# The Seductive Land of Carbs

# The Seductive Land of Carbs

## How to Avoid Carbobesity and Carbo-Gut

Find *your* carbohydrate tolerance. We all have one.
Determine the amount and type of carbohydrates that
best fit your heart, metabolism, and GI tract.
Carbohydrates to Fit You

Cindy H. Carroll, MS, RD, RN

BB Well Publishing
Bedford, MA

Published by
BB Well publishing
Bedford, MA

**Disclaimer:** This book focuses primarily on carbohydrates. Many other nutrients in food and factors in life, which have not been discussed here, influence our health, including the use of supplements, exercise, stress management, and so on. Please do not rely solely on the use of this information to treat or diagnosis any health or medical condition, physical or mental, that you may have, nor use it to replace consulting a medical physician. This book does not replace a medical appointment.

ISBN: 978-0-9907523-0-1

Book design and production by Bookwrights
Printed in the United States

# Contents

# Acknowledgments

Many thanks to the following people for their support and assistance.

My parents, who, although no longer living, taught me that I own my goals in life and it is up to me to complete them. I am forever grateful for their love and guidance.

To all of my clients, from whom I am continually learning as they allow me the privilege to step into their lives while they work at making difficult lifestyle changes. This book is really for you.

To my husband, Marcus, for his understanding and patience with my finally writing a book. To my two talented boys, Brendon and Ben, of whom I am most proud. Even though they really didn't know what I was doing until they saw the cover, I'm grateful for their continual support. Also, thanks to all three for being my IT department.

To my business coach, Marjorie Geiser, who quickly figured me out. Because of a severe injury that took me out of commission for many years, one of the first things I told her when I began working again was that I wanted to write a book. Within a few short months of working with Margie, I wrote a book. She's been a wealth of knowledge and a wonderful positive role model.

To my expert readers who helped confirm the accuracy of information and ensure ease of reading: Denise Barra, MS, RD, CDE, a kindred spirit in nutrition and someone who has always been ahead of the nutrition curve; Dianna Weikel, faculty member at the University of Maryland Dental School and University of Maryland Cancer Center; and Jane Wiggins, PhD, professor of anatomy and physiology, Middlesex Community College, Bedford, Massachusetts.

To Bob Land, as no book should be published without a copyeditor's eye. Thank you for your expert attention to all the details that scare so many of us.

To Mike Pabian for being my quick go-to copyeditor when I needed one.

To Mayapriya Long at http://www.bookwrights.com for the final typesetting and layout, and her ebook knowledge. Her expertise and professionalism were invaluable, especially for a first-time book author.

To a special photographer, Sue Bruce. Visit her website at www.suebruce.com.

To Bambang Suparman Ibrahim at Crowdspring, who helped design the cover. His image caught my eye right away, over many other talented designers. Who can't relate to a forkful of steaming pasta?

# Preface

I realize that searching for nutrition information can be a slippery slope. The Internet brings the words "search" and "nutrition" to another level. For those of you who have searched for anything nutrition-related online, it's a big world out there; the Wild West comes to mind. New frontiers were discovered in the Wild West, however. The beauty of technology and the Internet allows you to be a more sophisticated and informed consumer and also provides an easier venue for clinicians like me to educate. When used at its best, technology can be a win-win. I hope this book can also do that for you.

I'm a nutritionist/registered dietitian and a registered nurse. Early in my career I practiced as a sports nutritionist; then I switched gears and became more interested in functional/integrative medicine and its distinctive approach to health and disease. It has become my framework in assessing and caring for my clients, and now there's no going back. I believe it is the future of health care.

My approach recognizes that likely all of your history has brought you to where you are today, not just one event. Functional/integrative medicine is an approach to medical care that considers a person's entire history from birth to the present, while also recognizing that all of the systems in our bodies work together. Every person's body and needs are truly unique.

Functional medicine is as evidence-based and grounded in science as traditional medicine. Most practitioners—physicians, nurses, nutritionists, and so on—who employ it use both. It's really not outside-the-box thinking but is quite methodical and logical. Part of the reason that functional medicine makes so much sense to me as a nutritionist is that it strongly recognizes the enormous role nutrients play in just about every pathway in our body. If this thinking is outside the box, then our medical box is way too small! My nursing education and experiences have further cemented my belief in the importance of a more holistic approach to health care. We are not made up of separate parts and systems. Our body parts talk to each other and it's best if we listen.

Medicine has so much conflicting information, and sorting through it to best suit your needs can be tricky. What I learned twenty-five years ago is not necessarily the best advice today, particularly regarding carbohydrates. But being educated under the conventional medical model, I understand how the medical system works—its pros and cons. My functional/integrative medicine education has better taught me to look at the whys of disease versus just treating the symptoms. Functional medicine calls this looking more "upstream" versus "downstream." This approach has helped me look at research more objectively to figure out what it is really showing and not be afraid to follow my own path and instincts. This book follows my own path with what I believe about carbohydrates based on the past and current science and my over twenty-five years of counseling clients for a variety of medical conditions.

A word about dietitians: My nutrition education is primarily in the areas of nutritional biochemistry and sports nutrition, but my degree has also given me training in psychology. Interestingly, one outstanding factor in a dietitian's education and experience, perhaps unknown to most people, is that we've been trained to be diet detectives and to help you change your behavior. Both of these skills allow us to see what you are really eating as well as your lifestyle patterns. It's easy to just say we eat too much or the wrong foods. Finding that pivotal spot where you can change your behavior with food is key to your success. Having listened to thousands of diet histories of how people eat, these coaching skills regarding your behavior are invaluable to me in supporting you to be well.

It doesn't do you or me much good, however, to help you change your behavior if I'm giving poor advice. Today, many dietitians are more progressive in their education and experience beyond the food pyramid. We have to be because the public demands it. All nutrition professionals, including dietitians and nurses need to work hard at staying abreast. Few things stay the same in life. Medical information is constantly changing, especially in nutrition. The interest in credible nutrition knowledge is exploding, but nutrition research can't keep up. In the meantime, what is a person to do? Keep searching! If you doubt the information that health professionals give you, don't ignore your instincts. If you've never questioned any medical information given to you, perhaps it's time to start. Ultimately, caring for *you* is most important. The study of nutrition in medicine and its far-reaching effects on your body is just scratching the surface. You need to keep searching for what feels best for you.

For more information on functional medicine, please refer to the Institute for Functional Medicine's website at https://www.functionalmedicine.org and the Dietitians in Integrative and Functional Medicine's website at http://integrativerd.org.

# Introduction

The purpose of this book is to help you navigate the land of carbohydrates and determine your carbohydrate tolerance. Everyone has one. Determine what yours is and you will enter a much healthier state of living and avoid what I call carbobesity and carbo-gut.

Part of my incentive to write this book is that, over the course of my career, it's become clear to me that despite all of the diabetes and low-carbohydrate dieting information available, the public still does not have a clear understanding of what carbohydrates are, which foods contain them, or their effects on the body. For many, the carbohydrate world is black-and-white: either you eat a lot of them or you don't.

This book is not a diet book or a cookbook or even a specialty book on a particular medical condition. It is a book on the nutrient group known as carbohydrates, to give you a better understanding of the paths they take in the body after we eat them, their implications in a number of medical conditions, and their effects on health and disease. I talk about two distinct paths that I believe carbohydrates follow in our bodies and two systematic approaches to tailor your carbohydrate intake to fit your individual needs. You may find yourself firmly planted on one path, or you may see that both paths apply to you. The truth is that the paths overlap, which is one of my reasons for writing this book.

Carbohydrates are enticing and seductive nutrients. Whether you struggle with weight gain, high blood sugar, high blood pressure, or GI complaints, finding your carbohydrate tolerance will help all of them. (Note: "GI" and "gut" are used interchangeably throughout this book to refer to the gastrointestinal tract.) No, carbs are not a panacea or magic bullet, but they are so connected to so many systems in our body that it's nearly impossible to not see health improvements when you adjust your intake. By determining the amount and type of carbohydrates that work best in your body, you can determine how much of the other calories work best for you, too.

Appendix 1 includes sample days and summary charts for various food groups to help address short- and long-term goals while you lower your carbohydrates, a list of foods you can eat, and some handy resources for more information. I've never been big on making meal plans. They sound nice and tidy; you're given a written menu of exactly what to eat, and what could be wrong with that— right? Brainstorming meal ideas and making grocery lists are great exercises, and I do both with clients all the time. But giving a precise meal plan for you to live by never teaches you how to make choices. You don't need to become a nutritionist, but you do need to get the gist of what the main nutrients are, where they are in food, and what they do in your body. Couple that with behavior coaching and you are armed for life with skills to make your own meal plans.

This kind of information can be tedious, so I tried to keep the text short—short chapters and key takeaways at the end of each one. My experience is that the people who love this stuff will finish the book and probably be looking for more. But for those of you who are curious and just want to cut to the chase, this book is made for you. It includes enough detail to empower you but still allow you to finish easily. To keep the reading straightforward, references appear at the end of the book.

Most of all, I want you to become familiar with this nutrient group and think about your own body and how you feel after you eat carbs.

So . . . relax, sit back, and allow me to introduce you to this special class of nutrients of which we've all become so fond: carbohydrates.

# Part 1

## How Did We Get Here with Carbohydrates?

# 1

# Carbohydrates and Culture

arbohydrates are the rock star of nutrients. We have a love/ hate relationship with them. They even have their own abbreviated name: "carbs"—sort of like Madonna, Cher, and Lady GaGa—although carbohydrates are definitely a bigender nutrient. Society may perceive protein to be a more "manly" nutrient, and carbs mentioned more frequently in female conversation. Actually, men and women both can have carb issues. Former NFL quarterback Dan Marino's Nutrisystem commercials refer to many of their dishes as "man food," but you can be sure those meat-based meals provide plenty of carbs.

For as long as I've been studying nutrition, carbohydrates have been the main event. The Internet is loaded with information, and low-carb eating is now the premier carbohydrate show. As food fads come and go, this may be one fad with legs, albeit with several caveats.

Early in my education and through the 1980s when I was a sports nutritionist, carbohydrates were the pillar of the nutrition community. Particularly for athletes, they were and still are thought to be the primary nutrient to fuel muscles and power the brain. A low-carb diet was akin to nutritional snake oil and disastrous for any athlete. This was also the time when many heart disease studies were being used to form the framework of our national heart disease prevention guidelines. Today we still maintain the belief that fat is bad and will make you fat, cholesterol is bad, and both contribute to heart disease. Plenty of research now challenges these assumptions. Looking at much of the original research more carefully reveals many holes in their hypotheses.

Understanding the various impacts that carbohydrates have on

3

the body could fill several large textbooks. There is a lot to cover, and this book doesn't do it all. It gives you, however, a jump start to understanding the basics of this nutrient group and provokes you to pay attention to how your body handles them. In other words, the book guides you to *find your carbohydrate tolerance*. It is designed to highlight the benefits and perils of carbohydrates and how to go about closely examining your own body type and medical history, so that you can figure out what carbohydrates are the right fit for you!

## Key Takeaways

1. The medical community is looking differently at the roles and effects of carbohydrates on our body, even in the sports nutrition world.
2. Fat and cholesterol are not the villains in heart disease that they have made out to be. It's time to introduce the other players.

# 2

# Can We All Just Agree, Please?

When it comes to carbohydrates, you can find "experts" in both extreme camps: the strict vegans who say to eat only plants and no animals, and the no-carb advocates, who encourage eating only animal meat and their products. I believe the most support lies somewhere in the middle, with some guided rules.

To make a point early on here, I'd like you to consider reading from a growing list of authors listed in the Appendix who are actually putting their research into practice. Many are traditionally trained physicians or other specialists who have crossed over to use other approaches because they've become uncomfortable caring for clients with treatment that doesn't work. These people are not simply passionate nutrition advocates who decided to create a website and start giving advice online. They are medical physicians, specialists, well respected in their fields, who care for people every day and who have seen what works and what doesn't. I give them credit for following what they believe and not being anchored to the so-called accepted wisdom.

Although none of the books are flawless, their overall premise is sound. Listen to their overarching message; don't become too critical with the finer points. Quite frankly, medicine and science don't know the answers to many of the finer points, and no one plan works for everyone.

Interestingly, the authors of many of the books recommended in Appendix 4 cross all disciplines; they include cardiologists, endocrinologists, neurologists, sports nutritionists, and biochemistry researchers, yet their message is quite similar. They all speak extensively about the risks of excessive carbohydrates.

5

## Science Is Never Perfect

Unfortunately, when the media picks up on a diet or idea that strays from the U.S. government's My Plate guidelines, the promoters of such concepts are often harshly criticized because they are not following the herd. Of course, some practices are clearly unsafe and unwise to follow. But medical pioneers who operate outside the mainstream often make positive medical changes occur faster. I once read a commentary by a physician criticizing another physician's guidelines on gluten for people without celiac disease. People with celiac disease cannot digest gluten, the protein found in wheat, rye, and barley. Gluten's effect on people who do not have celiac disease is controversial—more on that later. The physician's concern was that some doctors take research data and extrapolate diet advice from the data that is not evidence based because it does not relate to the original research question that the author posed. In other words, the study didn't answer the original research question, but raised other questions.

Keep in mind that nutrition research is hardly flawless and takes years to complete. Many variables influence data and are difficult to sort out. Much research uses retrospective data, looking back on people's eating patterns and trying to make associations. Unless the subjects are actually housed in a research facility and monitored, their dietary intake is speculative; relying on subjective food recalls is not foolproof. I learned this firsthand while working on my graduate thesis at Massachusetts General Hospital.

And then sometimes, after years of work, the results don't answer the original study question—perhaps for many reasons—but often raise many more questions. Trusted, evidence-based nutrition information with double-blind, placebo-controlled studies is hard to come by. When I say "trusted," I mean studies with no ulterior motives or incentives such as drug profits. Evidence-based medicine at its best includes not only sound research but also clinical expertise and input from the patient; after all, patients are the owners of their body. Peer-reviewed, evidence-based research is still the gold standard for all practitioners, but we would be ruling out an awful lot of eating options for people it we waited for traditional evidence-based research to catch up, because food is not illegal nor does it require a prescription. Find a qualified nutrition expert who can sort through the layers of information out there and help you decide which eating pattern is safe and best for you.

## The Food Industry and My Plate

The presence of carbohydrates in the American diet has grown disproportionately to their benefit. The U.S. food industry, partially led by grandiose government guidelines, has targeted fat as the culprit to our health woes, which has catapulted our country into a carbohydrate feeding frenzy for a good twenty-plus years.

Perhaps the best part of Robert Lustig's book *Fat Chance* is his documentation of the political motives for maintaining carbohydrates in the base of the food pyramid. He so nicely outlines why as a society we remain stuck in the food pyramid muck. Regardless of our status quo, the result has been epidemic obesity, diabetes, and other chronic diseases, as well as food addictions. It is easy to understand why if you understand how carbohydrates work in the body.

You may ask why the government doesn't change its guidelines if all of these experts see it differently. You've heard the saying, "You can't fight city hall"?  In fact, many physicians and researchers are trying to improve the government guidelines, and I believe they will succeed one day, because the science is there. The "My Plate" guidelines improve upon the food pyramid but still don't put carbohydrates in the clearest, healthiest perspective. Although the government and its guidelines may be slow to change, you still can make the changes to your own lifestyle that feel the best for you. At some point, you just have to do what you believe in and what is right for your body. You will know it when you do it!

For a short time I followed the herd and counseled lower fat and higher carbohydrate intake for my clients. But my instincts and growing beliefs were not comfortable practicing this way. It was becoming quite clear that what works for one person does not work for all.

## Key Takeaways

1. A lot of carbohydrate camps are out there, ranging from strict vegans to low-carb advocates, and the Internet has lots of people

giving advice because the field of nutrition is a free market. Tread cautiously but be curious. Before you decide which camp you fall into, understand how carbohydrates affect your body.

2. More and more medical professionals are reviewing the scientific literature as well as assessing their own clients and believe reducing carbohydrates is a smart approach to reducing many health disease risks. Read a variety of opinions from different medical disciplines and question your caregivers.

3. The role of fat and cholesterol in foods and their effects on your health is evolving. They are probably not the villains that they were made out to be. Not all guidelines are fit for everyone.

# 3

# Your Genes and Carbs

Carbohydrate tolerance is influenced by epigenetics—that is, not just your genes but how your lifestyle and environment influence your genes. Eating too many carbohydrates if your body wasn't designed to leads to what I call *carbobesity* and potentially GI distress, or *carbo-gut*. No, these terms are not in the dictionary—yet! But they paint a picture that I see based on years of observing my clients' eating patterns.

We can't change our genes, but we can change some of the things that may trigger them to turn on certain processes. This is not a book on epigenetics, but know that it is a huge field in medicine. Knowing about your epigenetics may help you gain more control by being aware of positive and negative triggers for your body.

How food can have such an impact on all of our bodily systems is an overwhelming concept, because the number of vitamins, minerals, and phytochemicals—in addition to protein, fat, and carbohydrates—in foods and their multiple roles in our metabolism is immeasurable. Phytochemicals are compounds in foods that are thought to have many beneficial properties and give foods their color. Foods have thousands of different phytochemicals. We have identified just a fraction of them.

To put this in perspective, think of HTML, JavaScript, and every other computer code out there and mix them all up; that's how complex food's impact is on our bodies, especially considering our own unique DNA and unique blueprint of organisms that live in our bodies. Nutrigenomics is a field of medicine that examines food and its effects on our genes. Research is showing that food is basically an *epigenetic modulator*, meaning that it can influence our DNA for good or bad. So whether you choose the honeydew donut or the honeydew melon each morning, either way, they may be making their way to your DNA.

Some behavior specialists believe that most people don't care or want to know this kind of information, the *whys* of what's good or bad for us in life. Don't lecture me, right? Just tell me what to do. "Au contraire," I say. In my twenty-five years of counseling, I've seen enough people make short- and long-term changes to learn that it *is* the whys of what we should or shouldn't do in life that ultimately help people make necessary long-term changes to their lifestyle. I have seen too many clients make a nutrition appointment because their physician told them to, request a diet plan, and then believe, *Okay, I'm good.* Your daily world is literally surrounded by carbohydrates, making the whys of finding your carb tolerance all the more important.

Some people want the short version, and some like the long, detailed version. This book is somewhere in between. Your eyelids won't close, but you're still armed with enough information to get started. Later, I walk you through how to determine your own carbohydrate tolerance based on your medical history and lifestyle.

## Key Takeaways

1. We all have a tolerance level to carbohydrates depending on our genetic makeup, medical history, and lifestyle.
2. The field of nutrigenomics is showing that nutrition and food may be epigenetic modulators in our body. In other words, what you eat may turn your genes on or off.
3. Nutrition and how it affects our body is anything but simple. There are too many variables in food, the organisms in our body, and our genes to know how they all work together—but we are learning.

# Part 2

## Some Nutrition Basics

# 4

# Meet the Three Macronutrients

To help put carbohydrates in perspective, I like to remind my clients that there are three main nutrients or macronutrients in foods, from which we derive calories: *carbohydrates, protein, and fat.* Foods differ with how much of each they contain. Helping to frame my beliefs about these three nutrients was the work I did on my graduate thesis on protein in the 1980s while at Massachusetts General Hospital, as well as authoring a book chapter on protein in the 1990s. What I learned researching those projects helped form my foundation for understanding the necessity of protein in our diet, and my views and instincts have not changed.

Protein is the only nutrient for which our needs are based on preserving our optimal lean body weight. Our most basic need to survive depends on protein preserving that lean weight and for structure and repair purposes. It is the bedrock of building the house to make cells, enzymes, hormones, and tissues. Our need for protein is based on our need for individual amino acids to help all of that construction to occur.

We only need so much protein to perform this role. Any excess is excreted or used for fuel or energy, not protein's best job, especially if it takes from our own body stores of lean tissue. I calculate a rough protein requirement for all of my clients based on their optimal body weight, usually between 1.0 and 1.5 grams/kg (kilogram) of optimal body weight, occasionally going as high as 2.0 grams/kg of body weight. The research on protein utilization has not changed and still holds steady, recognizing the need for not skimping on protein. The only sound research that supports not upholding this protein range is with end-stage renal and liver disease. Otherwise, too little protein may well do more harm than good. Be careful when characterizing a diet as high protein; there is a difference between *high protein* and *optimal protein*.

Fat has significant roles, too, including helping prevent deficiencies of vitamins A, D, E, and K. Fat is structurally a part of every one of our cell membranes and plays a hefty role in allowing our cells to communicate. Certain fats, such as conjugated linoleic acid found in dairy products, may offer protection from cancer as well as cardiovascular and nervous system benefits. Our nervous system and brain are largely fat and water and rely on the right fats in our diet to function optimally. The best fat in food also has anti-inflammatory properties. We need fat!

Unlike protein, our need for fat and carbohydrates is largely based on our energy needs, although these two nutrients behave much differently in the body. There is no established or truly agreed-upon medical "need" for starches, sugars, and so on, as there is for fat and protein, although we may have a requirement for fiber in the large intestine to ensure the presence of certain protective nutrients and to keep things moving along.

Carbohydrates are more the loose cannons or fireballs that carry greater health risks. They can take you down the road to *carbobesity* and GI complications: *carbo-gut*. Before we figure out your carbohydrate tolerance, let's look more closely at this nutrient group and understand what carbs are, what they do, and what they can do for you. One size does not fit all.

## Key Takeaways

1. Protein is the most important nutrient to help us build and protect the structure of our body.
2. We have a definite requirement for fat—for example, for energy, structural purposes, cell communication, and immune protection.
3. We have no medically agreed-upon requirement for carbohydrates. We need it for energy and probable GI benefits. Excess carbs can harm the body. Everyone's needs are different.

# 5

# What Are Carbohydrates?

Indulge me here in just a little chemistry, because some basics are needed for you to become a bit friendlier with carbohydrates and truly identify them if you passed them in the street. Chemically, carbohydrates are varying chains of sugar molecules containing carbon, oxygen, and hydrogen, ranging from sugars with one sugar molecule called *monosaccharides* to two sugar-linked molecules called *disaccharides* to multilinked sugar molecules called *oligosaccharides* and *polysaccharides*. Carbohydrates in biochemistry are synonymous with *saccharides*, the Greek word for "sugar."

*Monosaccharides*, the one-linked sugars, are the end of the road—the simplest carbohydrate—and cannot be broken down into smaller carbohydrates. Examples of monosaccharides include *glucose, fructose,* and *galactose*. These sugars are found in varying amounts in foods, such as fruit and milk. If you love fruit's sweet flavor, you can thank the monosaccharides. Most fruit is really approximately only 50 percent fructose, and the other 50 percent is glucose. Some fruits have slightly more fructose than glucose, and the ever-so-common, man-made high fructose corn syrup is about 55 percent fructose and 45 percent glucose. As we will see later, higher fructose consumption may affect the body in different ways.

*Disaccharides* are two linked sugar molecules and include *sucrose* (glucose and fructose), better known as "table sugar," and *lactose* (glucose and galactose), the sugar found in milk products.

*Polysaccharides* are termed *complex carbohydrates* because of their many sugar links and are found in foods we call "starches"— the hard-to-stop-eating stuff: pasta, potatoes, rice, crackers, and bread. Other polysaccharides such as gums and pectins may also show up added to food (more on these later).

To digest any sugar, we must have the necessary enzymes to break their chemical bonds. The enzyme our body makes to accomplish this task is perfectly matched to the sugar, like a key in a lock. Enzymes identify themselves by ending with the letters "ase." The example you may know best is *lactase*, which unlocks or breaks the link in the sugar, *lactose*, found in milk products. If these enzymes are absent or fewer, digestive life can become, well, not so fun.

*Fiber* is also a type of polysaccharide but is the nondigestible form that humans cannot break down to absorb. Fiber provides roughage to keep your gut moving and your bathroom visits regular. It also provides fuel for those bugs in your gut to form nutrients, such as vitamin $B_{12}$ and healthy short-chain fatty acids. Some fibers also may help you maintain a more stable blood sugar. It has become popular practice for manufacturers to add their own fiber to foods that did not originally have them, a seemingly good marketing strategy given our old-school love of fiber. Common sources of added fibers are inulin, chicory root, and FOS (fructooligosaccharides).

To add a few more names to the list, starch can also be categorized into two main types: *amylose* and *amylopectin*. Amylose is linear in appearance, makes up about 20 percent to 30 percent of starch and contains more of the beneficial resistant starch that is harder to break down (more on that later, too). Amylopectin may raise your blood sugar more, contains more branches, and is the more prevalent form in our food supply.

*Sugar alcohols* are just as their name suggests: alcohols made from sugars. They occur naturally in foods but are also added as thickeners and sweeteners. They are not associated with tooth decay but can raise your blood sugar and cause a commotion in your gut. Recognize sugar alcohols by the "ol" at the end: *maltitol, erythritol, sorbitol,* and *mannitol.*

We'll talk more about FODMAPs later, but for now just know that they are fermentable short-chain carbs, including oligo-, mono-, and disaccharides, found naturally and added to food and a handy meal for gut organisms.

Have I lost you? Hopefully not! If you are not a science person, too many of these "ase" and "ide" words may have you yawning, but please don't go. Some of these words appear on food labels and you should recognize them as carbohydrates, at least being aware of what they are.

A List of Carbohydrates as They Might
Appear on a Food Label

Amylose, amylopectin, monosaccharide, disaccharide, polysaccharide, oligosaccharide, starch, corn starch, wheat starch, fiber, dextrose, sucrose, fructose, glucose, galactose, lactose, maltose, maltodextrin, inulin, chicory root, FOS, tapioca starch, potato starch, flax, sorghum, gums, and pectins.

# Key Takeaways

1. Carbohydrates are varying chains of sugar molecules containing carbon, oxygen, and hydrogen. They come in varying lengths and names.
2. Recognize the various names of carbohydrates on a label because they may be added to a food that did not naturally contain them, thereby increasing the total carbohydrate content of that food.
3. Remember that *saccharide* is Greek for "sugar."

# 6

# Where Do Carbs Live?

Foods have different mixtures of all three nutrients—protein, fat, and carbohydrates. When I talk with my clients about the foods with the most carbohydrates, I point to the ground. Carbohydrates primarily are found in anything grown from the ground, with the exception of most dairy products. Since milk and yogurt contain the sugar lactose, they contain carbohydrates, too, but they also contain protein and fat. Technically, meat and fish contain carbohydrates as well, because of the glucose stored in their muscles, but for the purpose of the measurable carbohydrates that show up on a food label, I am not counting them in our carb-containing food lists.

Although some nutrition camps consider milk controversial, check out how plentiful it is in all three macronutrients: carbohydrates, protein, and fat. Dairy also contains the beneficial fat known as conjugated linoleic acid, as well as a form of calcium that our bodies may prefer. Not all dairy products contain equal amounts of lactose. Milk contains the most. Be careful of added sugars, especially in yogurts and dairy drinks that raise the carbohydrate content. Read the label.

Whole milk is a good example of a food that contains all three macronutrients: protein, fat, and carbohydrates. The box below shows a typical food label for whole milk.

18

**Whole Milk Food Label**

Serving size 1 cup (8 oz. or 240 ml)
Total calories 150
**Total carbohydrates 12 grams**
Sugars 11 grams
Fiber 0 grams
**Protein 8 grams**
**Fat 8 grams**
Saturated fat 5 grams
Trans fat 0 grams
Polyunsaturated fat 0 grams
Monounsaturated fat 2.5 grams
Sodium 120 grams
Potassium 380 grams

The remaining foods that contain carbohydrates are grown from the earth. Let's get familiar with them. (We'll talk more about gluten later, but for now, know that it is a protein found in wheat, barley, and rye grains.)

## Foods Grown from the Ground

**Gluten-free grains.** Amaranth, arrowroot, bean flours (garbanzo, fava, Romano), buckwheat, corn, fava beans, flax seed, garbanzo beans (chick peas), hominy, mesquite flour, millet, montina flour, nut flour and nut meals, oats, pea flour, potato flour or potato starch, quinoa, rice (all forms), rice bran, sago, sorghum flour, soybeans and soy flour, tapioca (manioc, cassava, yucca), teff flour.

**Gluten-containing grains.** Barley, bulgur, chapatti flour (atta), couscous, dinkel or spelt, durum, einkorn, emmer, farina, farro, fu gluten flour, graham flour, kamut, malt, matzoh meal, orzo, rye, seitan, semolina, textured vegetable protein, triticale, wheat (bran, germ, starch), any gluten containing sourdough flour.

Have I forgotten any? Maybe, but hopefully you're getting it.

**Sugar (various forms).** Yes, sugar is grown from grass and doesn't come from a box. Types of sugar include agave, beet sugar, brown sugar, syrup cane-juice crystals, caramel, carob syrup, corn syrup, dextran, dextrose, fructose, fructans, glucose, inverted sugar, lactose, maltose, maltodextrin, mannitol, turbino sugar.

Don't forget other sources of sweet-tasting treats that don't sound like a chemistry lab: maple syrup, molasses, and honey. The sweet taste means it contains carbohydrates. *Fat and protein do not taste sweet.*

**Tree foods.** Anything grown from a tree, including apples, pears, oranges, and so on, and the juices made from them.

**Vine foods.** Anything grown from a vine, including grapes, berries, tomatoes, melons, and the juices made from them.

**Vegetables.** All of them—asparagus, artichoke, beets, broccoli, carrots, cauliflower, celery, green beans, leafy greens, onions, radishes, squashes . . .

**Legumes.** By definition, legumes are fruit or seeds from a plant—red, black, white, and garbanzo beans; lentils; and peanuts, too.

**Potatoes and yams.** White, red, and sweet—all types of tuberous root vegetables.

**Tree nuts.** Did you know that tree nuts are actually a hard-shelled fruit? This group includes almonds, Brazil nuts, cashews, chestnuts, filberts/hazelnuts, macadamia nuts, pecans, pistachios, and walnuts.

Perhaps the biggest light-bulb moment for my clients when it comes to carbohydrates is realizing which foods contain high amounts of carbs. Often clients say to me, "You mean fruits and vegetables are carbohydrates, too?" Indeed they are, but unlike grains, they are much more nutrient-dense.

Remember: *Carbohydrate-containing foods are foods that are grown from the ground. If it's a plant, vine, or tree, it contains carbs.*

---

**One last look:; A Summary of Foods with Carbohydrates**

Dairy: Milk, yogurt, ice cream, cottage cheese, kefir, some
soft cheeses
Any form of sugar
All grains
All fruit
All vegetables
All legumes
All nuts

---

# Read the Label

Many carbohydrates added in processing are disguised with
other names. Some foods that did not have many carbohydrates to
begin with end up with more carbohydrates because of these added
ingredients.

When reading a food label for carbohydrates, in addition to
looking at the ingredient listing, look for *three numbers plus the serving size.*

- Total carbohydrates in grams
- Sugar in grams
- Fiber in grams

The sugar and fiber numbers should add up to the total carbohydrates. Some labels have a number for *net carbohydrates*, which
is the total number of carbs minus the fiber. When counting carbs,
some diets count only the net carbohydrates. We'll investigate fiber
more later, but I tend to use the total carbohydrates number. Many
foods have fiber added that is not naturally part of the food, trying
to lower the carbohydrate total via the net carb route. As we will
soon see, fiber isn't an automatic free pass; tread carefully with net
carbs, too.

Every gram of carbohydrate contains 4 calories. For example, a
typical slice of bread may have 15 grams of carbohydrates and 80
calories per serving:

15 x 4 = 60 calories; thus, 60 of the 80 calories are from
carbohydrates.

I cannot underestimate the value of checking the serving size. I recently had a client who started drinking protein drinks, thinking they were low-carb. The bottle claimed, "Sugar-free." But upon closer inspection, each serving had over 20 grams of carbohydrates from maltodextrin . . . and the bottle contained two servings. You can do the math.

Let's practice a little on reading the label of one of my favorite foods, dark chocolate. Keep in mind that these numbers vary with the manufacturer.

Serving Size: ½ bar (43 g) of dark chocolate
Servings per container: 2
**Calories: 220**
Total fat: 17 grams
Saturated fat: 10 grams
Cholesterol: 0 mg
**Carbohydrates: 17 grams**
**Dietary fiber: 5 grams**
**Sugars: 11 grams**
Protein: 4 grams

The total amount of carbohydrates in half a bar or one serving is 17 grams. There are 5 grams of fiber and 11 grams of sugars. Surprised about the fiber? (I'm so proud of dark chocolate for naturally having fiber.) If we add the fiber and sugars, it comes pretty close to the total carbohydrate number, though not exactly. Manufacturers round off numbers, so for them it's close enough to the total of 17 grams to account for all of the carbohydrates.

To get the net carbohydrates number, subtract the fiber from the total carbohydrates.

17 grams − 5 grams = 12 grams net carbohydrates

# Key Takeaways

1. Certain dairy products naturally contain carbohydrates because of lactose.

2. Other than dairy, foods that naturally contain carbohydrates are grown from the ground and include fruits, vegetables, grains, legumes, nuts, seeds, and sugars.

3. Read the label to determine the amounts of total carbohydrates, total fiber, net fiber, and total calories in a food. Most importantly, *read the serving size!*

# 7

# How Much Lives Where?

## *What's A Lot of Carb?*

This chapter offers a general guideline of the carbohydrate content of various food groups. These numbers are really rough, so it's always best to read the label for the most accurate information. The best foods, however, often don't have labels with ingredients listed. Fresh broccoli or apples, for example, have no label, although perhaps they deserve a label to give them more recognition than the boxed foods we buy.

Interestingly, the nutrition guidelines of the American Diabetes Association consider foods with fewer than 20 calories and 5 grams of carbohydrates to be "free." Twenty calories is not many calories, and 5 grams is certainly fewer carbohydrates per serving than many other foods.

We'll talk about the pancreas later, but it's the most important organ when it comes to metabolizing our zealous carb intake. Let's just say for the moment that the pancreas probably doesn't consider these foods "free," especially with multiple servings.

Look closely at the serving size. It's a rare, usually conscious effort to eat just one-third of a cup of cooked pasta or a quarter of a large bagel. We even chastise people when they do eat such portions, with comments like, "Is that all you're going to eat?" In reality, those people are the smart ones!

## Grams of Carbohydrates per Food Group

*Grains/Breads/Cereals*
(Each of these foods equals about 15 grams of carbohydrates)
1 slice bread
¼ large bagel
6-inch tortilla
⅓ cup cooked pasta or rice
¾ oz. unsweetened, cold cereal
½ cup oatmeal or other cooked cereal
3 cups air-popped popcorn
4–6 crackers
½ English muffin or hamburger bun

*Milk/Dairy*
(Each of these foods equals about 12 to 15 grams of carbohydrates, except when otherwise noted)
1 cup milk
¾ cup or 6 oz. unsweetened plain or Greek yogurt
6 oz. flavored yogurt made with low-cal sweetener
1 oz. feta cheese—1.2 grams carbohydrate
1 oz. blue cheese—0.7 gram carbohydrate
1 oz. cheddar cheese—0.1 gram carbohydrate
1 Tbsp. cream—0.5 gram carbohydrate
1 Tbsp. butter—0 gram carbohydrate

*Fruits*
(Each of these foods equals about 12 to 15 grams of
carbohydrates)
1 small piece of fresh fruit (4 oz.)
½ medium fruit (apple, banana)
½ cup canned fruit in own juice
1 cup melon-honeydew or cantaloupe
1½ cup watermelon
¼–½ cup fruit juice
2 Tbsp. dried fruit
1 cup raspberries
1¼ cup strawberries

1 cup blackberries
¾ cup blueberries

*Vegetables*
(Each of these foods equals about 15 grams of carbohydrates; ½–1 cup = 5 grams)
3 cups raw vegetables
1½ cup cooked vegetables

*Starchy Vegetables and Beans*
(Each of these foods equals about 15 grams of carbohydrates)
¼ large baked potato (3 oz.)
½ cup potato, peas, or corn
½ cup cooked beans/legumes (garbanzo, kidney, or black beans)
1 cup winter squash
⅓ cup cooked cassava, yam, taro
⅓ plantain (green or yellow)

*Sweets and Snack Foods*
(Each of these foods equals about 15 grams of carbohydrates)
1 Tbsp. sugar or honey
2 very small cookies or 5 vanilla wafers
2-inch-square brownie or cake without frosting
½ cup ice cream or sherbet
2 Tbsp. light syrup
4–6 crackers
8 baked chips, potato, pita

*Source*: 2014 Diabetes Care and Education Dietetic Practice Group

## What's a Lot of Carbs?

Many people count calories and have a general understanding of what's a lot of daily calories. For example, 3,000 calories a day is probably too many for the average sedentary Joe or Jane, and 500 calories a day is not enough. But when it comes to the amount of carbohydrates eaten every day, most folks don't have a context for that number.

We'll talk soon about how the type of carbohydrate may offset the total count, and as you read this book these numbers will start to make sense. From my years of observation, I can report that most Americans eat more than 250 grams of carbohydrates a day—easily. That number has gone higher over the last decade.

When people are bingeing, or just want that "one last piece," or eat half the box of pasta and then a row of Oreos or crackers . . . that's easily 250 grams of carbohydrates, and often upward to 500 grams or more per day. One row of crackers may range from 80 to 100 grams. The Atkins diet and other low-carbohydrate diets usually mandate 50 grams a day or less. Endurance athletes and others like Michael Phelps may eat as much as 500 to 600 grams of carbohydrates a day, but are you exercising like Michael Phelps? Are you built like Michael Phelps?

The science behind how many grams of carbohydrates are best for you is evolving. Low-carbohydrate diets and diabetes research have helped spur some of this interest on the actual number of carbs eaten every day. As we will see, these numbers may deserve more respect.

---

**Carbohydrates in a typical American meal**

| | |
|---|---|
| 2 cups pasta | 90 grams |
| 1 cup spaghetti sauce | 24 grams |
| 2 slices of Italian bread | 30 grams |
| 1 cup non-starchy vegetables | 10 grams |
| 1 piece fruit | 15 grams |
| 1 cup milk | 12 grams |

**Total      181 grams carbohydrates**

---

## Grab a Pencil: Take the Carb Wake-Up Call Challenge

Hungry yet? Hang on, and soon we'll get to how much and what you *should* eat. First, though, I'd like you to reflect on what you *do* eat. Grab a pencil and paper and write down two days of eating. I call it the **Carb Wake-Up Call Challenge**.

Let one day be a typical day, including all of the good and not-so-good foods you eat. Importantly, include the amounts, regardless of how big or small they may be. Be honest! Then write down a day of eating when you forget about the nutrition gods and you just want to eat without any rules. Remember again to include the amounts. Your lists should show a typical day of eating and a worst-case day of eating.

Now look up the amounts of carbohydrates for each food and add up your total for each day. Use the label first, if you have one, or my guidelines in the previous chapter. You can also consult some online references, including www.calorieking.com or the USDA National Nutrient Database at http://www.nal.usda.gov. Even just Googling the type of food will show you the carbohydrate content along with other nutrient information. Add up your total carbohydrates for each of the two days. If you have the fiber content, add that up, too, and subtract it from the total carbohydrates number. You'll then have a net carbohydrates number and, more importantly, a total fiber intake number. (As I mentioned earlier, I rely more on the total number of carbohydrates.)

I realize that you may want to skip this exercise altogether, but I promise you that the act of looking up the carbohydrates and keeping this record will make an imprint on you and deliver a jolt of reality that you will not forget. So many of my clients have taken this challenge and not only been blown away by how quickly carbs add up in a day, but for the first time in their lives they feel like they had a confident sense of how to manage what they eat, with positive results.

When you've listed and tabulated your two days, hold onto those numbers. We'll use them later to see where you stand with meeting your carbohydrate tolerance.

## Key Takeaways

1. Read the food label and pay attention to how many total carbohydrates are in the foods you eat. Become familiar with which foods have more, and always check the serving size!

2. Because carbohydrates are so abundant in foods, especially processed foods, it is easy to eat a lot of carbs quickly.

3. Take the Carb Wake-Up Call Challenge. Count how many carbohydrates you eat for two different days. How can you learn what is best for you if you have no clue what and how much you usually eat?

# 8

# Carb's Vocation: From Food to Gluco–Glyco What?

## *What Do Carbohydrates Do for You?*

Energy! The primary role of carbohydrates for humans is to provide energy—to supply the glucose (sugar) molecules to our cells to form ATP (adenosine triphosphate), the fuel that allows you to jump out of bed every morning. You may be thinking, *Wait a minute. Carbs do other things, too, such as provide taste, comfort, and pleasure.* The food companies have recognized the taste, comfort, and pleasure roles all too well and have many of us wrapped around their little carb fingers.

Nature intended carbohydrates primarily for energy. Hunter/gatherers would forage berries and other plants when these foods were in season to add to their body stores and to provide a source of energy that they could convert to glucose. Prior to wheat harvesting and modern agriculture, carbohydrate foraging was not a 365-days-a-year, three-to-six-meals-a-day activity. It was truly seasonal, depending on where you lived.

Wheat harvesting was not only our modern society's introduction to a regular higher carbohydrate intake but also provided a reliable income for farmers. Wheat has become one of the main ingredients in the American food supply. Some aboriginal cultures have seen the advent of modern carbohydrates in their diet only in the last 100 years. Some cultures still don't ingest modern carbs, and I say, good for them!

## Gluco–Glyco What?

Humans convert carbohydrates from food into glucose, which our cells use for energy (ATP). We also store carbohydrates from glucose in the form of glycogen (a form of polysaccharide) in our liver and muscles for later use. A 150-pound man stores about 320 calories worth of glycogen in his liver, and his muscles store about 1,400 calories (athletes store more). Making more glucose than you need sends it to the fat storage bank.

In the sports nutrition world, the more fit you are and the more carbo loading you do, the more glycogen your muscles can store. When we need glucose for fuel, we call upon it from our glycogen stores in our liver or muscles. Our liver is usually filled to the brim from our frequent daily dining on pasta, pretzels, bagels, and such.

One limitation in this process, however, is that only muscles can use muscle glycogen. Organs such as the brain can't knock on muscle's door and say, "Hey, could you send over some glucose, glycogen, or whatever you've got?" Can't be done. The liver, however, is quite generous in doling out glucose from glycogen to organs in need, such as the brain. Later we'll discuss what our organs use for fuel, but many experts believe that excessive carbohydrates—particularly in an unfit body—may make it easier to store fat and harder to use the body fat stores we do have for fuel.

If you do lots of endurance exercise, you need more carbohydrates than sedentary folks, but research is showing that even endurance athletes probably don't need the volume of carbohydrate loading I learned about back in the 1980s.

## Key Takeaways

1. Carbohydrates' main role in the body is to provide glucose to our cells to make ATP—the fuel we use for energy.
2. We store carbohydrates in our muscles and liver as glycogen.
3. Access to carbohydrates wasn't always so easy. Humans did not evolve with carbs at every street corner.

# 9

# Fiber's Vocation

Aside from energy, the next best thing carbohydrates provide is fiber, except that most of the carbohydrates we eat today are refined, lacking in fiber. And because many of us have disturbed GI tracts, when we do eat fiber, it may make matters worse. In a perfect carbohydrate world, carbohydrates should offer soluble and insoluble fibers and resistant starches that maintain proper motility in the GI tract, help form the perfect stool, and provide proper fuel for the organisms in the large intestine—assisting them in forming such things as the short-chain fatty acids and B vitamins that are important to our health.

Insoluble fiber does not dissolve in water and is usually found in the outer bran layer of whole grains. This type of fiber helps move things along and propels the gut's contents forward.

Soluble fiber actually swells in water, forming a gel. Food sources include oat bran, barley, nuts, seeds, and beans. If you can picture this gel mass in your gut, you can understand how it actually slows digestion—helping you feel fuller, possibly preventing blood sugar spikes, as well as helping trap toxins and other substances in the gel, carrying them out during your next bathroom visit. Oatmeal and barley both contain beta-glucan, a special polysaccharide that research is showing may be related to lowering cholesterol and blood sugars.

Resistant starch is a form of indigestible starch and is grouped as another type of fiber, not to be confused with mainstream fiber. Resistant starch is naturally found in foods and is also chemically changed to resist digestion. Research demonstrates that resistant starch may help increase those short-chain fatty acids in the large intestine, but may be problematic if fermented by the bugs in your small intestine, thus contributing to excessive bloating and gas. Examples of various forms of resistant starch include uncooked potatoes, unripe bananas, high amylose corn, seeds, unprocessed whole grains, and legumes and some grains that have been cooked, then cooled.

## Refined Redefined

Ian Spreadbury, a researcher at the Gastrointestinal Disease Research Unit at Queen's University in Ontario, nicely describes some of this carbohydrate stuff. His research reveals that, up until the era of modern agriculture, our ancestors ate a variety of carbohydrates—what he calls *cellular carbohydrates* with intact cell structures. On the other hand, we are largely eating *acellular carbohydrates* that no longer have such form.

Acellular carbohydrates are basically carbohydrates that manufacturers have poked, prodded, and refined. Their form has been disrupted; they have lost their integrity. One might argue that foods that have been manipulated from their original form are foreign to our gut. Moreover, refined, processed carbs offer far fewer nutrients than whole foods.

A quick and simple way to identify a product with refined or acellular carbohydrates is that it comes in a box or package. The more ingredient listings on the label, chances are the more refined or processed it is. Those foods with the longest ingredient listings have really been poked and prodded.

Eating mostly processed carbohydrates may confuse our balance of organisms in the gut, encouraging overgrowth in the wrong places, which we talk about later. When the wrong organisms show up where they shouldn't, they can change the body's pH to be less protective, as well as produce gut-damaging toxins. Refined carbohydrates also raise your blood sugar, which we soon discuss in depth.

No question, this change in players changes the show. And when you add other factors such as medications and over-the-counter drugs to treat a variety of ailments—acid blockers; antidepressants; statins; anti-inflammatories, including both nonsteroidal (NSAIDs) such as Advil and steroidal such as prednisone—the GI population may change even more. This is a pivotal point of carbohydrate tolerance, and we return to it later.

## How Much Fiber?

The following table shows the Institute of Medicine's Daily Dietary Reference Intake for fiber. These recommendations work best in an optimal gut world. The reality for many people is that optimal fiber intake is often determined by trial and error. Because science shows fiber largely to be a positive influence on our bodies, these guidelines are still good goals.

Grams of Fiber per Day

| | |
|---|---|
| Men age 50+ | 30 |
| Men age 19–50 | 38 |
| Women age 50+ | 21 |
| Women age 19–50 | 25 |

## Key Takeaways

1. Fiber is an indigestible form of carbohydrates that may have many health benefits. The two main types of fiber, insoluble and soluble, behave differently in the body.
2. Determining the right amount of fiber for you may be tricky because of GI issues, but adequate fiber is still a good goal.
3. Resistant starch is a form of carbohydrate that may have health benefits.
4. Refined carbohydrates or acellular carbohydrates have been manipulated by manufacturers and have many negative effects when eaten, including changing gut health and raising blood sugars. Any carbohydrate in a box, can, or package—and especially with a long ingredient list—is more processed and refined.

# 10

# Glycemic Index and Glycemic Load

The glycemic index is a measure of how fast a sugar in food elevates your blood sugar. The glycemic load gives more attention to the quantity of food needed to raise blood sugar. Carbohydrates are the nutrient group that contains the most sugars and the most variety of sugars. Some foods may have a high glycemic index, but the amount to produce a significant increase in blood sugar may not be what most people consume. Watermelon is a good example of having a higher glycemic index but a lower glycemic load. The highest glycemic index score for how quickly a food raises your blood sugar is 100.

Other factors in food—such as protein, fat, and fiber—also affect how quickly and how high your blood sugar may rise. Overall, to help prevent obesity, cardiovascular disease, and diabetes, some research supports eating lower-glycemic-index foods (55 or less), such as legumes, nuts, seeds, steel cut oats, and barley. If you eat foods with a medium glycemic index, between 56 and 69, then eat them with adequate protein, fat, and fiber to slow your blood sugar rise. Medium-glycemic-index foods include processed grains, soda, Gatorade, and even some whole grains. Yes, you read that correctly: some grains can raise your blood sugar as much or more than soda. Overall, for some people it may be best to limit high-glycemic foods with a score greater than 69, including potatoes without the skin, many breads, and sugars.

Keep in mind that everyone is different. I have seen many type 1 diabetics and some type 2 diabetics whose blood sugar elevates even with steel cut oats or oat bran. Of course, the amount or portions of foods make a difference, too. Blood sugar is a big deal. It becomes an important marker for your health. You'll see why soon.

The University of Sydney's website, http://www.glycemicindex.com, is a great resource for the glycemic index and glycemic load of various foods.

## Key Takeaways

1. Glycemic index and glycemic load refer to how quickly a food raises your blood sugar. Glycemic load takes into account the quantity of food.
2. Other factors affect how quickly a food raises your blood sugar, including portion sizes and protein, fat, and fiber in the same meal.
3. Research suggests that eating lower-glycemic-index foods and limiting higher-glycemic foods may have health benefits.

# Part 3

# The Effects of Carbohydrates on the Body

# 11

# Carb Addict?

## *Do You Have an Achilles Carb?*

bsolutely! Before we discuss carbohydrates' effects on the rest
of the body, it's important to know that carbohydrates affect
our brain, mood and behavior. This topic is too extensive to delve
into deeply, but it is important to keep in mind. Carbohydrates,
especially sugar (sucrose), can be addictive. They fulfill the scientific requirement of an addictive substance, which includes causing withdrawal symptoms when removed. Experts do not all agree
on carbohydrates' effect on mood and behavior, and a number of
biochemical pathways are probably involved, including hormonal,
as well as the competition of amino acids across the blood-brain
barrier.

Carbohydrates activate the brain reward centers by boosting
levels of neurotransmitters in the brain when consumed in certain
ways, which may help improve our mood and sleep but also may be
linked to negative moods. Because of changes in these neurotransmitters, including serotonin and dopamine, we can have a love/
hate relationship with sugar and other carbohydrates. The medical
community is starting to recognize this connection. Many parents
intuitively already know that their children's Jekyll/Hyde transfor-
mation after Halloween is not just compliments of the full moon.

Research also shows that the proteins in gluten in wheat products attach to the opioid receptors in the brain, potentially giving you that same gotta-have-it feeling that some opioid drugs give. These proteins are called *opioid peptides* and are classified as *exorphins*. Exorphins may sound familiar. They are similar to *endorphins*, the feel-good chemical our body makes, but instead we get exorphins from outside the body.

It becomes a slippery slope when our likes, desires, and wants in life turn into a need or requirement. Sorry to say, but our bodies don't require sucrose, although we may wish they did. Because of its addictive properties—and especially combined with fat, salt, and caffeine—sugar nicely fits that addictive substance model. Add the effects of insulin, which we talk about in the coming chapters and unfriendly organisms, (see more later in the book under "Your Gut on Carbs") and our addictive tendencies may become worse. Most people don't think of food this way, but just as my first biochemistry professor in college told me, "Food is chemicals." Food can have drug-like effects on our body; prescription not required.

According to the American Psychiatric Association's *DSM IV-TR* criteria for substance abuse and dependence, at least three of the following seven requirements must be present for a substance to fit the addictive substance model. (Note: A new version of the DSM, *DSM-V*, was released in May 2013. This new version does not separate substance "dependence" and substance "abuse" but rather gives a single diagnosis, "substance use disorder," based on nearly the same criteria combined. A minimum of two to three criteria is required for a mild substance use disorder diagnosis, while four to five is moderate, and six to seven is severe.)

Although recognizing binge eating disorder as a diagnosis, *DSM-V* still does not formally include food in the addictive substance model, but many believe this change is on the horizon. The model does include caffeine.

Beyond its nutritional value, food becomes a double-edged sword. Food is not all about providing energy and nutrients. Food is pleasurable, spiritual, and enjoyable, as it should be. We celebrate with food. We give with food and we reward with food, but we also punish with food. The accompanying box presents some statements about addictive substances as mentioned in *DSM IV-TR* criteria. Be honest: Do you see yourself in any of the statements as they apply to your intake of sweets and starchy foods?

**Do Sweets or Certain Carbohydrates Cause
Any of the Following for You?**

1. Building a tolerance—requiring more to get the same effect.
2. Withdrawal—physical and psychological signs when substance is removed.
3. Bingeing or use of substance in larger or larger-than-intended amounts.
4. Persistent desire or attempt to cut down or quit; craving or seeking; interference with life; use despite negative consequences.
5. Involvement in chronic behavior to obtain the substance, use the substance, or recover from its effects.
6. Reduction or abandonment of social, occupational, or recreational activities because of substance use.
7. Use of the substance even though there is a persistent or recurrent physical or psychological problem that is likely to have been caused or exacerbated by the substance.

## Identify Your Achilles Carb

When the negative physiological or social effects of carbohydrates outweigh the mood boost or pleasurable role we may get from them, it's time to look at your carbohydrate tolerance and find a different balance. Do you have a favorite carbohydrate that runs your life—an Achilles carb? Many people can eat hundreds of grams a day of their Achilles carb. It may be bread or pasta, rice or sweets. If you consistently overeat your Achilles carb, learn how to eat *mindfully* instead of *mindlessly.* Mindful eating is all about awareness and intent and takes practice. Restricting certain carbs cold turkey or setting clear boundaries may help you make long-term changes. An example of a clear boundary is one serving of bread a day or 1 cup of pasta once a month.

We will be discussing two systematic approaches to finding your carbohydrate tolerance, but if you are vulnerable to addictive tendencies, all the more reason to find your carbohydrate tolerance and live by it.

## Key Takeaways

1. Carbohydrates change the neurotransmitters in the brain, including serotonin and dopamine, which affect our mood.
2. Carbohydrates, when consumed in certain ways and by certain people, fit the definition of an *addictive substance*, although they have not yet been officially categorized as such by the American Psychiatric Association's *DSM* criteria.
3. Identify if you have Achilles carbs and set boundaries around them.

# 12

# Carbohydrates Leave a Trail
## *Let's Walk Down Two Paths*

By now you know I'm leery of lots of carbohydrates . . . and my family even used to call me, "the bread lady." Carbohydrates are not a "free" group of foods that have no effect on our body. I believe they are a class of nutrients we need less than we think and potentially take the greatest toll on the body when eaten to excess, rather than fat or protein, as we have been led to believe. In fact, we have come to overeat carbohydrates so much, that it is often at the expense of fat and protein, spinning many folks into essential fatty acid and protein deficiency and imbalances. When it comes to carbohydrates, one size does not fit all. Understanding your carbohydrate tolerance may well be your ticket to health and preventing the diseases of *carbobesity* and *carbo-gut*.

What happens when humans are exposed to much higher levels of carbohydrates than ever before? Carbohydrates cause damage from going down two distinct paths, and these two paths separately and together can wreak havoc with your health. Everyone is a bit different on how these paths work, depending on your genes and lifestyle.

## Path #1

Carbohydrates exert a great demand on the pancreas to produce insulin. Insulin is a hormone the pancreas makes that is absolutely essential to our existence, but if consistently oversecreted, even in small amounts, insulin can contribute to inflammation, diabetes, aging, and possibly cancer. Too many carbs may also direct our body away from burning our fat for fuel.

## Path #2

Carbohydrates provide fuel for gut organisms and can disrupt your unique gut world: the bacteria, archae, viruses and yeast inside you—your *gut microbiome*—creating what's called a *gut dysbiosis*, or as I call it, *carbo-gut*. All foods may affect the type of organisms in the gut but sugary foods and starches may have a profound effect, contributing to overpopulation in the wrong places. Under the right conditions they may also help lead organisms out of the large intestine, higher up into the small intestine, stomach, and even esophagus. Combine this with antibiotics, antacids, NSAIDs such as Advil, or other triggers such as food poisoning, pregnancy, or stress, and certain carbohydrates can compromise your digestive tract and potentially your immune system.

\* \* \*

Both of these paths that carbohydrates follow can be somewhat subtle, happening behind the scenes, creeping along for years, until *bam!*—your body reaches a threshold. You may ignore many signs along the way, but at some point, your body will tell you in no uncertain terms that your *carbohydrate threshold* has been reached—whether it is outright diabetes, insulin resistance or prediabetes, weight gain, IBS, ulcerative colitis, fatigue, or all of the above.

The insulin and gut pathways of carbohydrates are becoming better understood, but they are still spoken of separately, as if they are mutually exclusive, which is probably incorrect. The organisms living in our gut may well be related to insulin resistance. Microflora or microbiome research is showing that the gut organisms are different for lean people than obese people, and the type may affect insulin regulation.

To take it a step further, your sweet tooth may be encouraged by too much insulin and your unique gut bugs—and you thought you were in control of your life, right? Well, you can be, but in a way, your hormones and the creatures inside you are at the wheel, too.

*Million-dollar question:* I don't know the correct answer, but this book is an attempt toward exploring an expensive question: *How many carbohydrates are necessary to help maintain a healthy gut before they promote excess blood sugar and insulin production?* And if you had to choose, which is more important: a healthy blood sugar and lower insulin levels or more gut protection? I'd rather not choose, but the negative health implications of high blood sugar and insulin levels are well understood. Less is known about the gut and immunity; medicine is just beginning to understand its magnitude. Some people are so metabolically resistant that they require ketosis (see in chapter 28) to shift out of insulin resistance. My hope is that most people, especially if they begin the practice early enough in life, can find a carbohydrate balance that is low enough to keep blood sugars and insulin healthy, while high enough and of the right type to maintain a healthy gut, too. One may well be related to the other.

Let's now look at the two paths separately of how carbohydrates may do some of their damage.

## Key Takeaways

1. Carbohydrates affect the body in many ways; including taking two paths after we eat them. *Path #1:* Raise blood sugar, thereby placing a demand on the pancreas to secrete insulin. *Path #2:* Provide fuel for gut organisms. With a healthy gut, this fuel may have benefits, but many factors can tip the imbalance, causing problems.
2. Factors that may tip your carbohydrate tolerance to intolerance include: medications, certain medical conditions, stress, a sedentary lifestyle, and visceral belly fat.

# Path #1

## Your Heart and Pancreas on Carbs

# 13

# Cardiovascular Disease, Type 2 Diabetes, and Metabolic Syndrome

## *Who Dun What?*

We are trapped with a misinformed mentality about cholesterol and fat in food, as well as an emotional and physical attachment to carbohydrates. But a medical paradigm shift is in the making, and it can't come too soon. Many in the scientific community now view as largely bogus the targeting of fat and cholesterol as health demons. The pioneers of this emerging view remind us that cholesterol is not a disease, but rather a necessary component of every cell and therefore necessary for life. In fact, more and more research cites the risks of cholesterol levels that are too low. Largely, we balance our production of cholesterol with what we eat. With the exception of people in the extremes (people who have total cholesterol well over 300 mg/dL), the total cholesterol number is of less value, unless we know exactly what the LDL and HDL fractions are made up of both in quantity and type, especially the oxidized LDL, as well as other lipid components. Oxidized LDL is more inflammatory and carries greater health risks. But most physicians do not gather this information.

Inflammation is at the root of heart disease and many other chronic illnesses. Cholesterol may be found at the scene of inflammation but largely does not *cause* the inflammation; other things do, including the ever daily overabundance of insulin. This is not a book on cholesterol, but the long-held medical view of the lipid hypothesis' and its role in heart disease is showing its holes. Science has a lot to iron out with these views, but excessive carbohydrates—especially low-nutrient carbohydrates—fuel the problem.

We understand now that saturated fat in food is not a culprit either; it's really more a neutral to slightly inflammatory fat. Its potential inflammatory characteristics are probably much more a result of being in the presence of too much insulin—an outcome of eating too many carbohydrates. Most research on the inflammatory nature of saturated or any fat does not factor out the carbohydrates eaten with those fats. Also remember, some saturated fat helps form beneficial short-chain fats in the large intestine, which is a good thing. And eating fewer carbohydrates may help us burn the saturated fat that we store in our body.

The research community is in agreement, however, that trans or hydrogenated fats found in some fast food and packaged, processed food are culprits. We have no need or requirement for this man-made inflammatory fat. The food industry, including fast foods, has somewhat kept up with this research and is using less hydrogenated fats in its manufacturing. Read your food label and limit foods with the word "hydrogenated" in the ingredient listing. I'll go one step further and recommend avoiding any highly processed fats or any man-made fat that is not naturally found in plants and animals. The key here is to eat fats that are "naturally found and minimally processed." If the fat has been processed or manufactured, it adds a risk, just as with any processing or manipulation of any food . . . to say nothing of the debate over genetically modified organisms (GMOs), from which most corn and soy products are made.

Vegetable oils oxidize easily and do not withstand high heat well, making them potential inflammatory agents in the body. The worst vegetable oils are from corn and soybean; less risky may be a high-quality cold-pressed sesame and peanut oil. Cold-pressed extra virgin olive oil and coconut oil are the two I recommend.

## Inflamed on Insulin

The most important thing to remember about carbohydrate metabolism is that carbs require insulin to enable the final product of glucose to enter the cell from the bloodstream. The pancreas works hard to maintain normal blood sugars. High blood sugars and the need for more insulin is the bane of excess carbohydrates' existence, at least for us humans trying to stay healthy and lean.

Insulin is an anabolic hormone, secreted by the beta cells of the Islets of Langerhans of the pancreas. Insulin helps to build muscle at the right times, while aiding the transfer of glucose to the cell. But it also unlocks fat cells to let excessive glucose in to be stored. So, insulin's job is also to help store fat. In a healthy, nondiabetic person and even with some type 2 diabetics, the pancreas is constantly secreting a low or basal level of insulin that is finely tuned with a number of variables.

Those pancreatic islets cells also contain alpha cells, which secrete *glucagon*, a hormone that raises blood sugar. It works with the liver in regulating blood sugar if the blood sugar is too low. This regulating of blood sugar falls under the *endocrine gland* responsibilities of the pancreas.

The pancreas is a busy beaver; it also has digestive responsibilities that fall under its function as an *exocrine gland*. Keep in mind that the endocrine part of the pancreas makes up only 1 to 2 percent of its mass. Far more of its mass goes to the digestive enzymes and juices made to break down food.

So we're asking a lot of this organ when we overeat in general, but particularly when we overeat carbohydrates. Insulin's frequent presence in our bodies because of the constant American flow of cinnamon buns, latte specials, and even just a bag of pretzels puts an ever-present burden on our pancreas and those precious beta cells to produce. After carbohydrates are broken down to glucose, what is not used directly for energy is either stored in the liver or muscles in the form of glycogen or stored as fat in adipose tissue. Insulin is necessary for all of this to occur.

Most carbohydrates enter the bloodstream the same way, from the small intestines. Fructose, however, is processed a bit differently after it reaches the small intestines by entering the bloodstream from the portal circulation of the liver. Fructose is stored as glycogen and fatty acids in the liver. Interestingly, research suggests that fructose isn't as readily chosen by muscles to make muscle glycogen as is glucose. Much research holds that too much fructose results in a fatty liver. Fructose can also be hard on the gut, which we'll get to later.

And where is the worst fructose found? My vote is high fructose corn syrup (HFCS). HFCS becomes a risky ingredient because it is contained in so many foods—including soda and refined carbohydrates—and thus increases your daily fructose dosage. The fructose in fruit at least has fiber and other vitamins and minerals. Some studies suggest that fructose doesn't create the same satiety signals that glucose does, possibly encouraging the "I want more" feeling.

If you do have a fatty liver, besides the name itself sounding like something the neighborhood bully might call you, the liver releases those fats called *triglycerides* into the bloodstream and makes your blood triglycerides number go up. Which foods in excess contribute to fatty liver and high blood triglycerides? The answer begins with a "C"—Carbohydrates, especially refined carbohydrates.

Since the start of my career, most fatty liver disease was believed to be from alcoholism or medications. But now we understand that elevated liver enzymes are also from excessive carbohydrates and abdominal obesity. So, the fat around your belly from excess carbs, not the fat in your diet, raises your triglycerides—a really important distinction.

The other risky part of eating a surplus of carbohydrates that result in high blood sugars and fatty liver is that it may direct fuel usage away from your fat stores. How any one person burns protein, fat, and carbohydrates as fuel is an individual matter, but research suggests that a fatty liver does not maximize your fat-burning ability. It may compromise your fuel usage away from burning the fat around your belly for fuel.

Fiber is the only type of carbohydrate that is largely indigestible and asks the least of insulin. Foods with more fiber typically produce less of a rise in blood sugar, provided that they are not loaded with other added sugars.

## Was It Meant to Be This Way?

The pancreas's production of insulin is complex and has a genetic component, so we are not all created equal with how our pancreas responds to carbohydrates or protein. Protein raises blood sugars, too, and therefore triggers insulin release—but not nearly like carbohydrates. Sports nutritionists recommend carbohydrates for athletes based on their sport and level of exercise, and then come up with an intake based on grams of carbohydrates per kilogram of body weight. These guidelines have nothing to do with the ability of the pancreas to keep up with this demand, but are purely from an energy perspective related to certain levels of exercise.

These guidelines assume that the pancreas will keep up because exercise helps with insulin sensitivity. I believe these guidelines are assuming a lot, particularly when it comes to surges of very high carbohydrate intake, especially high-glycemic carb consumption such as juices, sugar gels, candies, rice, and pasta. Perhaps more importantly, once they stop competing, many athletes keep eating carbs and don't ramp down their intake. The pancreas may then start to sputter.

## Let's Not Forget Leptin

Insulin is also friends with leptin, a word you've probably heard but don't know much about. Leptin is a hormone, released by fat cells. Its role is to tell the brain whether you have enough energy. When working correctly, leptin levels should coincide with when you are hungry and when you are not. Excessive insulin blocks leptin, signaling our brain to eat, even when our fat stores and blood glucose are at their proper levels. So, we eat when we don't need to. Sound familiar?

This disrupted leptin pathway is termed *leptin resistance*, much like *insulin resistance*, where insulin doesn't allow glucose into the cell. Leptin, though not deficient, is just not working correctly, so the brain keeps getting the signal from leptin to eat, when the body stores are fine. End result? Weight gain, obesity, and diabetes. What nutrient drives insulin? Yup, carbohydrates! Those refined, acellular, spineless carbs are leading you down the path to leptin and insulin resistance.

## Key Takeaways

1. Strong evidence questions the assumption that fat and cholesterol in foods cause high cholesterol and heart disease. Rather, research strongly shows that *inflammation* is a strong contributing factor to heart disease. Fat and cholesterol in foods are not direct causes of inflammation, with the exception of the harmful man-made trans fats in foods.

2. The pancreas bears a great responsibility in digesting and absorbing carbohydrates, especially in regard to its need to produce insu-

lin but also because of the enzymes it secretes to break food down. In susceptible people, excessive carbohydrates place a burden on the pancreas, potentially leading to insulin resistance.

3. All carbohydrates raise blood sugar and request that the pancreas release insulin. Chronic excessive insulin leads to insulin resistance and weight gain.

4. Leptin is a hormone that helps regulate appetite. Insulin resistance may lead to leptin resistance, which makes it harder to stop eating when you should, even if you want to.

5. Excessive carbohydrates, particularly excessive fructose such as in high fructose corn syrup, may contribute to fatty liver disease, thereby increasing blood triglycerides. It's the carbohydrates in food, not the fat, that increase blood triglycerides. High blood triglycerides are a risk factor for heart disease and metabolic syndrome.

# 14

# Do You Know What Your Blood Sugar Is?

For a society that eats so much of a nutrient group that dramatically affects our blood sugar and weight, few people know how many grams of carbohydrates they eat a day, and few know the number of the blood value it so intimately affects. We have been falsely focused on fat, believing that it drives up blood cholesterol and blood triglycerides. Blood sugar is only really examined when people are almost diabetic or clearly cross the road to diabetes. Blood sugar levels are a potential firestorm in our bodies. It's not uncommon for clients to tell me, "My doctor says my blood sugar is just a little high, just lose a little weight," or "I'm sure he checked it, but I don't know what it is."

Many factors aside from food affect our blood sugar, including medications, infection, hormones, fever, hydration, and visceral fat. *Visceral fat* is body fat that is stored within the abdominal cavity around important internal organs such as the liver, pancreas, and intestines. In excess it becomes belly fat that you can see in the mirror and watch grow and take a life of its own. Your clothes or belt loop are good measures to watch this fat change.

Visceral fat is sometimes referred to as *active fat*; research shows that it is almost an organ itself and plays a distinctive and potentially dangerous role affecting how our hormones function. Storing higher amounts of visceral fat is associated with increased risks for a number of health problems, including type 2 diabetes.

Check out the image of a gentleman with excess visceral fat at http://www.diabetes.co.uk/body/visceral-fat.html. The man on the right is probably secreting far less insulin to manage the same amount of food as the man on the left. Ladies, you are not exempt from visceral fat either. Women with apple figures often have excess visceral fat—larger waistlines than measurements for their hips and legs.

*A diet high in refined carbohydrates and low in fat is a prime cause of low blood sugar levels. Such a diet directs your pancreas to frequently release insulin, the hormone that helps to lower blood sugar.*

You may not even be aware if your blood sugar is elevated, but you probably know when it starts to fade. You may become a little jittery, weak, and headachy, and have mood swings and the desire to eat. Given the frequency and the types of carbohydrates we eat, the average American pancreas is on daily overdrive, keeping our blood sugars in a game of yo-yo and totally reliant on the next refined refueling. Proper liver function along with a healthy pancreas is important to help regulate our blood sugar. Youth and a somewhat healthy body can generally cover up all of this—for a time. If you've ever gone to your doctor for a checkup and he checks your fasting blood sugar and it's "normal," good for you! Your pancreas is producing what it needs to keep your blood sugar in check—at least for that moment in time.

Yet we really don't know how much insulin it took for you to keep your blood sugar normal because doctors don't usually check insulin levels. Many experts believe that physicians should be measuring insulin, since excess insulin can occur sometimes years before a high blood sugar shows up, but few do. The medical standard for normal fasting insulin ranges from 6 to 26 uU/ml (microunits per milliliter). This is what the textbooks say and what medical practice follows, when they test it. Also helpful is the insulin response to a glucose load by testing insulin after a standard oral glucose tolerance test. Some people may have normal fasting insulin levels but still produce too much after a meal.

*Try to picture this.* Your average insulin resistance curve starts out with you perhaps being a healthy lean or even slightly overweight but making enough insulin to match your carbohydrate intake. As your busy life entices you to eat more carbs and gain more fat, especially around your belly, the beta cells in your pancreas start pumping out more insulin to keep up. It may work for a time, keeping your levels normal, but eventually blood sugars will start to creep up and the fat around your belly will contribute to the insulin receptors in your cells to respond less to even greater amounts of insulin in an effort to carry glucose to the cell

So, your cells go hungry, your blood sugar stays elevated, and your pancreas is overworked. That's the inner workings of *carbobesity!* I wonder what the insulin levels were of the folks living on the little house on the prairie?

## What's a Normal, Healthy Blood Sugar?

By most guidelines, a fasting blood sugar of less than 70 mg/dl is considered *low blood sugar (hypoglycemia)*, and a fasting blood sugar greater than or equal to 100 mg/dl is considered *high blood sugar (hyperglycemia)*. A fasting blood sugar greater than 126 mg/dl taken on two occasions could equal a diabetes diagnosis. A few years ago, however, a new fasting blood sugar zone of 100 to 126 mg/dl was officially recognized as *prediabetes* or *insulin resistance*. Now a normal fasting blood sugar should be between 70 and 100 mg/dl.

What was the compelling reason for this change? Research was clearly showing that fasting blood sugar levels over 100 mg/dl are related to a higher cardiac risk, recognizing the inflammatory impact of what we thought was just a little elevated blood sugar.

Blood vessels have a permeability, too, much like the gut wall, which we talk about later. The most inside layer of blood vessels is called the *endothelium*, which has receptors and communicates with various parts of the body. The health of our endothelium is key to cardiovascular health. When blood vessels leak because of oxidation and inflammation, they become more permeable, allowing debris inside, over time forming what we know as plaque. Damage to our vessels really begins with damage to the vessel wall itself, not with the lumen or inside and the eventual plaque deposit.

Keeping your blood sugars normal helps prevent leaky blood vessels and plaque buildup. Plaque buildup is made up of not just fatty deposits but calcium salts and other ingredients. Unstable plaques that may dislodge are made of riskier or more inflammatory material. Just because vessel plaque contains fat doesn't mean the fat you ate caused it. High blood pressure, environmental toxins, and obesity all contribute. But you can also thank your refined, spineless carbohydrates and a high blood sugar for a good part of that inflammation.

We are better understanding now that our body doesn't really discriminate with the enemy when it comes to how it fights our battles. Whether it is a virus, stress, environmental toxin, or excessive sugar and other refined carbohydrates, our body responds in a similar way—with oxidation, inflammation, and some type of immune response. Cardiologist and blood pressure specialist Mark Houston of Vanderbilt University extensively studies the endothelium and cardiovascular health, and his research is on the forefront of how best to measure our risk, as well as what we need to do to change it. Check out his work at the Hypertension Institute of Nashville, http://www.hypertensioninstitute.com.

## Key Takeaways

1. Check and keep track of your blood sugar. A normal fasting blood sugar should be less than 100 mg/dl.
2. A high-carbohydrate diet, especially refined carbohydrates, is a prime contributor to high and low blood sugars because of the continual demand for insulin.
3. High blood sugar is a marker of inflammation and a risk for heart disease.
4. Visceral fat, especially around the belly, is a major contributor to insulin resistance. Excess carbohydrates contribute to excess visceral belly fat.
5. Check your insulin levels. Insulin levels can begin to rise years before your blood sugar becomes abnormal.

# 15

# Diabetes and Heart Disease: Two Peas in a Pod

Y ou can't have diabetes without cardiac risk. Likely, if you have heart disease, you have some level of insulin dysregulation or even prediabetes. Usually, once people hit their thirties or forties—and sometimes sooner if they are not active—they get a random fasting blood sugar measurement that creeps up over 100 mg/dl. Sometimes, their doctor will tell them, sometimes not.

I always advise my clients to ask what the number is and keep track of how many readings creep over 100 mg/dl.

A fasting or random blood sugar only tells what your blood sugar is at that moment in time. A one- to two-hour postmeal blood sugar has the benefit of revealing how adequate your body responded to that venti, triple mocha latte.

More of a storyteller, however, is hemoglobin A1C (HbA1C), a blood test that does not require fasting. It measures a protein in the red blood cell that reflects blood sugar levels over the previous three months. HbA1C is used to help diagnose diabetes and should be part of everyone's yearly physical, especially if you are over forty years of age; ask your physician. HbA1C measures glycation of proteins, a risk factor for other diseases as well as aging. Glycation gives some idea of the total inflammatory load of your vessels.

*An HbA1C of 5 percent is equivalent to the average blood sugar of about 100 mg/dl, and every 1 percent above 5 percent equals an additional 40 mg/dl increase in blood sugar. Diabetes is diagnosed as an A1C of greater than or equal to 6.5 percent. Aim for an A1C of 5.7 percent or less.*

## Hemoglobin A1C

| | |
|---|---|
| Less than 5.7 percent | Normal |
| 5.7 to 6.4 percent | Prediabetes |
| 6.5 percent or higher | Diabetes |

## Blood Glucose Level

| | |
|---|---|
| Less than 70 mg/dl | Hypoglycemia or low blood sugar |
| Fasting greater than or equal to 100–125 mg/dl | Prediabetes/hyperglycemia or high blood sugar |
| Fasting greater than 125 mg/dl on two separate occasions | Type 2 diabetes |
| Greater than or equal to 140 mg/dl at any time | Hyperglycemia or high blood sugar |

See also the information at http://www.diabetes.org/diabetes-basics/diagnosis/.

The U.S. Department of Health and Human Services estimates that about 80 million Americans, and probably more, have prediabetes. Much of my practice is made up of people with prediabetes. The good part of knowing you have prediabetes is that at this stage, it is most likely reversible with diet and lifestyle changes, without medications. The bad part: your pancreas is overworking, and your insulin is probably becoming less efficient. It may be the beginning of metabolic syndrome and is reflective of so many chronic disease risks. In other words, your body is saying, "*Helloooo*, please listen to me. *Please* don't ignore me or put me on hold. I'm trying to help you out here by giving you these red flags."

Here is a tidbit of information, buried in research but an exclamation point to this section of my book. The *New England Journal of Medicine* (see http://www.ncbi.nlm.nih.gov/pubmed/21366474 and http://www.ncbi.nlm.nih.gov/pubmed/16207847) reported on a study in which nondiabetic men with fasting blood sugars higher than 86 mg/dl had a greater risk of developing diabetes than those with values less than 81 mg/dl. Other studies have also shown that the risk of cardiac death is greater for those with fasting blood sugars greater than 85 mg/dl. Today, 85 mg/dl by any medical standard is considered a normal blood sugar.

You may wonder, *Why is she belaboring this blood sugar thing?* Aside from not smoking and maintaining a healthy blood pressure, maintaining a healthy blood sugar is perhaps the best thing you can do for your body and mind. Finding that sweet spot of blood sugar with the greatest health benefit is up to you. Too much sugar (glucose) in our bloodstream for too long a time is not good for our blood vessels. It is inflammatory and potentially sets up other inflammatory processes. The glucose then tells our body to try and compensate with extra insulin, a hormone that wasn't meant to be the driver all day. Then too much insulin potentially sets up the scene for too much fat storage and leptin resistance, making it mentally harder for you to make or want to make changes.

Ask your doctor what your blood sugar is and keep track of it. For some people, consider purchasing a blood glucose monitor and test your own blood sugar. Your blood sugar is a marker like your blood pressure. Few would argue against regularly measuring blood pressure. Blood sugar checking is a little more invasive, but for some people it is worth the knowledge.

## Polycystic Ovary Syndrome (PCOS)

A *syndrome* is a condition with a collection of signs and symptoms that may affect different organs. PCOS is a condition affecting a growing number of young women. Insulin resistance is a dominating characteristic of some forms of PCOS, something you might not suspect given that the name PCOS infers cysts on the ovaries. People with PCOS have a higher risk for type 2 diabetes and benefit from lowering their carbohydrates.

## What Are the Two Most Important Things to Keep Blood Sugar (Glucose) in a Healthy Range?

1. **Finding your carbohydrate tolerance.** A diet lower in carbohydrates with the carbs that best suit your body with adequate

protein and healthy fats puts less demand on your pancreas for insulin. Don't make your pancreas work harder than it has to.

2. **Exercise: Aerobic and resistance training.** As we age, if we don't limit carbohydrates, most people need more and more exercise to keep insulin levels stable. Resistance exercise helps the cells be more sensitive to the insulin that you do make so that glucose can better get into the cell. Aerobic exercise also helps insulin utilization. Plus, research shows that fitter athletes better use the triglycerides that are stored in their muscles. The fat is actually stored closer to their mitochondria, the powerhouse of the cell that allows fat to be converted to energy. Maybe it's nature or evolution rewarding you for moving.

## Key Takeaways

1. Diabetes is a major risk for heart disease. Usually you can't have one without some of the other. High blood sugar is a measure of inflammation of blood vessels throughout the body.

2. Hemoglobin A1C is measure of a protein in the blood that reflects blood sugar over the previous three months.

3. A diet lower in carbohydrates lowers the demand for insulin from the pancreas.

4. Aerobic and resistance exercise helps cells be more sensitive to insulin and improves insulin resistance.

# 16

# Carbohydrates and Cancer

I would be remiss if I didn't mention something about carbohydrates and cancer. Not enough research has been completed with humans on the effects of carbohydrates on cancer cells or the potential benefits on cancer of restricting carbohydrates. The American Cancer Society's guidelines do not mention lowering carbohydrates to prevent cancer, although its website mentions a variety of nutrient -dense foods that may behave as antioxidants and thereby possibly have protective effects.

Cancer and carbohydrates is not a new subject. Credible published nutrition research has been popping up since the 1920s when Nobel laureate Otto Heinrich Warburg discovered that cancerous tumor cells in the presence of oxygen use aerobic glycolysis to make ATP, followed by another pathway that produces high amounts of lactic acid (yes, a mouthful to process, but important information).

This discovery is called the "Warburg effect" and is a well-established trademark characteristic of most cancer cells. It sharply contrasts with the more efficient ATP-producing method that most normal cells take in the presence of oxygen. Normal cells with oxygen will utilize glucose (glycolysis) but then produce ATP via taking the pyruvate exit; remember the TCA or Krebs cycle? This generates more ATP and less lactic acid. Without oxygen, normal cells also utilize glucose in glycolysis and then take the road to lactic acid production. This produces far less ATP, but the process is quicker. The world record for the 100-meter dash would not be less than ten seconds if this was not true.

For normal cells, the anaerobic conditions (lack of oxygen) is what makes higher levels of lactic acid, but cancer cells opt for this less efficient means of ATP production even in the presence of a lot of oxygen. In fact, they use glucose up to 200 times more than normal cells of the same tissue. This was a pivotal discovery because it shed some light onto why cancer cells choose a seemingly inefficient pathway. Reproducing new cancer cells is probably the reason for their choice versus choosing an efficient means to produce energy.

As with everything in science, there is the complex version and the simple version. The science behind the pathways of glucose's association with the growth of cancer cells is complex, but the gist goes something like this: Most tumor cells rely on glucose as a fuel source to replicate—the Warburg effect. Easily available glucose via chronically elevated blood glucose levels may make this easier for cancer cells.

Many cancer cells have insulin receptors, and a growing body of evidence is associating high insulin levels, high insulin-like growth factor (IGF-1), and high blood sugars from prediabetes and type 1 and 2 diabetes with various cancers, particularly pancreatic, colorectal, and kidney cancers but also breast cancer. Research shows that chronically elevated blood glucose and high IGF-1 promote tumor growth and may worsen outcomes in cancer patients.

Research also shows that some tumors do not use ketones as a fuel source, making the state of ketosis a curious treatment option for cancer. More on ketones later, but they are produced when carbohydrates are less available in the diet. Some lab studies on animals show direct antitumor effects from ketone bodies themselves, possibly unrelated to other insulin and blood glucose alterations.

Many variables may be at play here, but one recurring theme is the role of high insulin levels and insulin-like growth factor in the proliferation of malignant tumor cells. One study by the University of Minnesota looking at 45,000 women demonstrated that women with diabetes had a 50 percent higher risk of developing colorectal cancer than those without diabetes.

Data looking at hunter-gatherers suggest that cancers were rare. In fact, cancers are really believed to be a more modern disease. Metabolic syndrome increases the risk for several cancers. The genes may be present in many people for various cancers, but we may be turning them on much more readily than did our ancestors (epigenetics). We have a number of options to turn genes on—stress, smoking, environmental toxins, poor diet, elevated blood sugars.

We know the formula to elevate blood sugars: a steady supply of the Western diet with lots of carbohydrates—complex and refined.

One more thought about our pancreas. The rates of cancer of this organ have increased in the last twenty-five years, coinciding with the dramatic increase in our intake of carbohydrates. The growing literature on carbohydrates' potential role with many cancers is evolving, but the association with pancreatic cancer is particularly important considering the aggressive nature of this type of cancer and the role this organ plays in digestion and glucose regulation. Maybe it's an indicator for us to look closer at the burden this organ must bear from our dietary imbalances.

## Key Takeaways

1. Far more research is needed, but cancer cells are fueled by glucose, possibly using a pathway that helps them replicate faster.
2. Cancer cells have insulin receptors and are sensitive to high insulin levels.
3. Research shows that people with diabetes have a higher rate of certain cancers.
4. A low-carb diet, including one that creates ketosis, may be a treatment option for certain cancers.

# Path #2

## Next Up: Your Gut on Carbs

# 17

# Meet Your Gut Microbiome

Once upon a time, it was believed that before we entered into this world, inside the womb, the human gut was untainted from bacterial exposure. More research, however, is showing that this notion is not true. Rather, the environment in which the fetus lives inside the uterus has its own microbiome associated with the placenta, amniotic fluid, and the meconium—that is, the "poop" of the fetus. When the soon-to-arrive baby takes a gulp during the ride through the birth canal, the child receives the first, more substantial inoculation of Mom's natural flora. The microflora of the fetus, infant, and the mother during pregnancy is under intense study in the worldwide microbiome field because this beginning period of a person's life is when the blueprint of organisms is developing. Research suggests that this blueprint is influenced by many factors, including the process of labor, hormonal changes, Mom's flora, Mom's diet, breast milk, and the mode of the child's delivery: elective or nonelective C-section or vaginal delivery.

This early state of microflora development may set the stage for health later. C-section babies have a gut flora closer to that of the skin because they build their gut flora initially more from their first surroundings, which is usually a hospital. C-section delivery is associated with a higher incidence of asthma and insulin resistance, possibly because those babies don't get that initial booster of Mom's good organisms to jump start their immune system. Some very recent research even suggests that swabbing a C-section baby with their mom's vaginal flora may have benefits. Also, supplementing premature infants with probiotics has been shown to help prevent an often fatal condition called *necrotizing enterocolitis*.

Keeping those "good organisms" balanced with the not so good is key to gut health, which may be key to overall health. The magnitude of the role that the organisms in our body play, particularly in the gut, in serving and protecting us is of great interest in the medical field. The National Institute of Health (NIH)'s Human Microbiome Project is just one of several global efforts studying the body's trillions of organisms. Our gut flora, primarily in our large intestine (colon), works on our behalf to make vitamins and nutrients, protect against infection and diseases including cancers and heart disease, and regulate our bathroom visits. Keeping inflammation at bay and our intestinal walls at an optimal permeability helps protect the rest of our body. Healthy gut microflora are very underappreciated servants, considering the many and important jobs they do.

*Gut permeability*, sometimes referred to as *intestinal barrier function*, is really important. The term is tossed around a lot, and we need to better understand its huge impact on our health. Excessive gut permeability is essentially the same as "leaky gut." The gut mucosal wall becomes more open, allowing things through that shouldn't go. Proper permeability allows the right nutrients to enter our bloodstream after they've been broken down.

Think of the small intestine lining as a gate that opens very carefully only for selected passersby. This gate is made up of cells called *tight junctions*, quite purposeful units of cell-to-cell connections. When that gate becomes damaged or looser with bigger openings, things pass through and enter the bloodstream that our body then has to deal with it. Some people do okay, but others interpret whatever passes through as an assault and on they may go to some kind of autoimmune disease.

Maybe the biggest question to be answered is, how does our gut mucosal wall lose its optimal permeability? We understand better now the events involved, but the sequence in which they happen is still debatable. The organisms that live in our GI tract probably run the show. And because up to 70 percent of our immune cells lay in the gut, when these orchestra leaders change places or move around, our gut plays different music.

## Gut pH

The coordination of how gut members work together to function efficiently is like a company with good internal communications, where all departments talk, listen, and pay attention. As in many parts of the body, the optimum pH for each part of the gut is important and helps create the environment for it to do its job correctly. The term *pH* can get people nervous because it implies chemistry and test tubes. I hear you, but understanding a little about your body's pH is just being smart. You might think twice before you do things that could change your pH.

Simply put, pH measures acidity or basicity (alkalinity) of a solution by measuring H+ (hydrogen) ions. A pH of 7 is neutral. Less than 7 is acidic; greater than 7 is basic. Our blood pH is tightly regulated between 7.35 and 7.45. The right pH is vital to life. The pH of various parts of the gut may change over a lifetime for a variety of reasons, including medications, diet, and gut flora.

## Key Takeaways

1. The fetus has its own world of organisms even before birth. Many factors influence an infant's gut world.
2. The organisms in our gut are key to gut and immune health.
3. Tight junctions are cell-to-cell connections in the small intestine mucosal wall that control gut permeability.
4. The gut members work together, and there is an optimal pH for each part of the gut. Changing the pH changes the health of the gut.

# 18

# A Quick Tour of the Gut

The gastrointestinal tract begins in the mouth, where we secrete enzymes along with our saliva that initiate the process of digesting food and signals other organs what is to come. In order to start the breakdown of food, saliva is slightly acidic, with a pH of about 6.8.

Then comes the esophagus, where the actual propulsion of food begins down to your stomach. Prior to this, food is hopefully helped out by your chewing and swallowing. But once past the mouth, food is on its own with your gut. The pH in the esophagus ranges between 4.0 and 6.0, slightly more acidic. With a pH of less than 4.0, esophageal tissue can be damaged or burned.

Onward to the stomach, mostly a holding tank for food, but it also churns up whatever we dump in it, preparing it to be better broken down before it alerts the small intestine to be ready for the next phase of absorption. The stomach also initiates certain satiety signals and has receptors for hormones. As we can all attest, the stomach can stretch and hold more food than we need at one time.

Here is perhaps one of the most important points of gut health. You know the saying, "There is a time and a place for everything." Well, the stomach is the time and place for a higher acid environment compared to the rest of the gut or body. The stomach produces hydrochloric acid (HCL), a strong enough acid to burn the skin. It also produces enzymes that help start protein digestion. HCL activates pepsinogen, the precursor enzyme to pepsin, the active enzyme, so that it can begin to dismantle the proteins we eat. If your stomach doesn't start breaking down protein because it has too little acid, it will pass the undigested food on to the small intestine. These undigested proteins are too big for the small intestine to do its job properly.

HCL also helps protect the stomach from invaders (a pH ranging from 1.5 to 3.0 in the lower stomach): very few organisms should live in the stomach. The pH may become slightly higher when churning up food. This acid not only helps kill off unwelcome guests that come in from our mouth that shouldn't go farther but also discourages organisms that may try and creep up from below the stomach.

A growing body of experts believe that adequate HCL is key to preventing overgrowth of bugs and maintaining proper gut balance, and that many people probably don't overproduce but rather underproduce gastric acid. Aging tends to decrease, not increase many of the gastric secretions including enzymes and stomach acid. Although heartburn or reflux of acid into the throat that gives you that burning feeling may seem like you are making too much acid, the culprit may more likely be the door or valve between your esophagus and stomach loses its ability to regulate itself properly and opens too easily for a variety of reasons. Normally, a low stomach pH between 1 and 3 signals that door to stay closed to keep acids contained in the stomach, but if the stomach is not producing enough acid, it doesn't fully get the signal to keep the door closed. So, underproduction of acid, along with other risk factors including obesity and the presence of certain irritating foods, may push that door open, releasing what little acid may be present. Both over- and underproduction of HCL present with similar symptoms, and without a careful assessment, treatment may be with unnecessary and potentially damaging antacid medication that may set the stage for further damage including nutritional deficiencies.

Actually, the argument some strict vegans make that humans are not supposed to eat meat becomes a fruitless point (pun intended). Whether you believe humans are herbivores or carnivores, we would not have evolved with HCL and pepsin in our stomachs ready to act on protein if they weren't to be used. They are there for a reason. No, we don't have as much HCL as other carnivores, but we're not supposed to eat a small animal at each meal. Remember: protein is the macronutrient that our body relies upon to build everything to survive. I strongly question evolution wanting to jeopardize the digestion and absorption of this nutrient. Our protein requirements are based on our optimal, lean weight and typically can be met by one to four ounces of animal protein at each meal.

From a nutrient perspective, it takes a very savvy vegan to be healthy. It can be done with the right body, but in the many years I've been seeing clients, it's a rare strict vegan who has adequate nutrient stores and muscle tone to stay healthy while aging.

One other point about the stomach: *gastroparesis* is a condition where the stomach muscles don't work properly to empty its contents in a timely manner. It produces bloating and potential shifts in blood sugar. One cause of gastroparesis is thought to be neurological damage to the vagus nerve that innervates the stomach muscles from diabetes and uncontrolled high blood sugars. How convenient that gastroparesis occurring in the beginning stages of digestion is related to other GI disorders as well as one of the greatest health risks we've spoken of at length, high blood sugars.

## Next Stop: Small and Large Intestines

Most of the nutrient absorption action takes place in the small intestine. It is not bugless, but the number of organisms should be much lower than in the large intestine. These organisms are strongly influenced by the foods we eat. The medical community has established a standard normal bug count for the small intestine.

The small intestine has three sections—the *duodenum, jejunum,* and *ileum*—and different nutrients get absorbed in different locations. The pH of the duodenum is about 6.0, a weak acid compared to farther down in the ileum, where the pH might be 7.0 to 8.5, a weak base. This pH helps balance out the acidic contents of the stomach and also helps the enzymes in the small intestine do their job properly without being harmed.

The mucosal wall of the small intestine is truly a work of art in terms of evolutionary design, selective to certain molecules, dictating traffic by using those tight junctions. It is vulnerable, however, to damage, and if injured can disrupt a lot of things.

Another cool but much underappreciated design feature of the small intestine is its migrating motor complexes (MMC). *MMC* is a movement that actually begins in the stomach and progresses into the small intestine to help propel its contents along, working to prevent stasis or backup. Research shows that properly operating MMC is a key toward preventing overgrowth of the wrong organisms. One key feature of MMC is that it needs adequate rest between meals for it to work properly, preferably a minimum of ninety minutes but possibly up to four to five hours may be better—not exactly the American way. The American grazing style, away from defined, structured meals and snacks, can hinder MMC from doing its job.

The organisms in the gut include some general characteristics that may determine their behavior. There are the *"healthy, normal organisms,"* and then there are the *"normal, but maybe not so healthy organisms,"* sometimes referred to as *opportunistic organisms.* Together these organisms are called *commensal organisms*—they co-exist, relatively peacefully. Then there are the *pathologic organisms* that can definitely do harm. The normal, but maybe not so healthy organisms are typically present but just not in high enough numbers to cause trouble. If the normal, healthy organisms become outnumbered by the normal, not so healthy and/or pathologic organisms, then trouble can ensue. Pathologic organisms usually occur because of infection from food poisoning or outside sources. Since the small intestine is where most nutrient absorption takes place, if it becomes overcrowded with too many organisms feasting on your carbohydrates, the nutrients available to you may be fewer. Examples of the typical organisms that can grow to excess include Bacteroides, lactobacillus, Clostridium, Streptococcus, Escherichia coli, Staphylococcus, Klebsiella, Enterococcus, and Klebsiella pneumonia. If diarrhea is present because of these excess organisms, malabsorption of nutrients can occur.

Finally, the large intestine, the neighbor next door to the small intestine, houses the most organisms—possibly over 500 different species. The main types of bacteria in the colon are anaerobes, and the most abundant bacteria are members of the genus Bacteroides, including gram-positive cocci, such as Peptostreptococcus, Eubacterium, Lactobacillu, and Clostridium.

The large intestine is the last stop in digestion and responsible for a lot too, helping to make vitamins and protective fatty acids. The pH of the large intestine ranges from 5.5 to 7.0, slightly acidic. And of course, this last stop makes the stool that we hopefully eliminate every day.

## Other Players

The GI track really starts with the mouth and ends with the anus. The pancreas, liver, and gall bladder are members of the digestive system, too, though not technically part of the alimentary canal or gastrointestinal tract. These organs play a big role in how nutrients in food are absorbed and how other toxins we consume are handled.

The pancreas contains digestive enzymes for carbohydrates, proteins, and fats—part of its exocrine gland functions—as well as cells to neutralize some of the acids in the stomach, making up most of the mass of the pancreas. If too little of these enzymes occur for a variety of reasons, digestion is impaired.

The liver makes bile that is stored in the gall bladder. Bile helps emulsify the fat we eat so that it is digestible. The liver also provides a systematic means of detoxifying pretty much everything that passes through it. Together these organs diligently work to keep up with our toxic lifestyles.

## Gut/Brain Connection

The enteric nervous system (ENS), sometimes referred to as the *second brain*, is a part of the nervous system that is actually embedded in the gastrointestinal tract starting at the esophagus and continuing all the way to the anus. This sophisticated system includes two networks of neurons that control digestive motility and blood flow. Key neurotransmitters are actually made in the gut, including most of our serotonin. Another sophisticated system called the blood brain barrier (BBB) is made of a capillary network with miles of blood vessels that nourish the brain and protect it from toxins. The interface and communication of these systems and what happens when parts become compromised is under intense study in medicine. Autism, Alzheimer's, and ADHD are just a few conditions with cognitive changes where research is examining their relationship with the brain/gut connection. The foods that we eat and their effects on the gut wall barrier may affect the brain and nervous system's health too. *Parts are not just parts....*The human body is connected.

# Key Takeaways

1. Digestion begins in the mouth and is synchronized between organs. If the stomach does not have enough acid to break down protein and protect its environment from hostile intruders, then further GI problems may arise.

2. Aim for a minimum of 90 minutes up to five hours between meals to allow MMC to do its job and keep organisms flowing out of the small intestine.

3. Most of the organisms in our gut should be in our large intestine, where they create beneficial fatty acids and vitamins, including vitamin $B_{12}$.

4. The liver and pancreas also play key roles in helping us digest and detoxify foods and their compounds.

5. The second brain or enteric nervous system is a complex network of neurons in the gut that interfaces with the brain and BBB. Many conditions that affect the brain and nervous system may be related to the health of the gut barrier and second brain.

# 19

# Rocket Fuel for the Gut

People have never eaten the amount of carbohydrates we eat today. In fact, most of the food we eat today is man-made carbohydrates. The average American's pancreas is pumping out insulin unmatched at any other time in history. A high sugar and high refined carbohydrate diet is rocket fuel for some gut organisms. Even the good carbohydrates, as we talked about, fuel them in the colon, which is okay. But if they overpopulate higher up, you have far less leeway for feeling good when eating carbohydrates. Many people with sensitive guts know how poorly they feel when eating even healthy carbohydrates, such as some fruits and vegetables.

## Fiber and Your Gut

I grew up believing that fiber is good. Nothing like a little fiber for what ails you, right? Straightens things right out. Well, sometimes it will, sometimes it won't. If you have a disrupted belly for whatever reason—celiac disease, Crohn's disease, ulcerative colitis, or IBS (irritable bowel syndrome), fiber may not straighten things out. In fact, it could bind things up.

The rules of fiber are difficult to follow because everyone's gut bugs are different, so what works to keep your best buddy regular may not necessarily work for you. Some fiber types may help diarrhea and constipation, and others may worsen them. Yet manufacturers keep adding fiber to everything, even foods that don't naturally have it.

Your unique gut print of organisms may determine how you will respond to fiber. Some fibers that are added to foods include galactooligosaccharide (GOS), inulin, and fructooligosaccharide (FOS) and are called *prebiotics*. Prebiotics stimulate the growth of organisms in the large intestine, not to be confused with *probiotics*, which are the actual organisms. If excessive organisms are in the small intestine, these fermentable foods can produce symptoms such as excessive bloating, cramping, diarrhea, or constipation.

Generally, the soluble and insoluble fibers found in fruits, skins of fruits, vegetables, seeds, nuts, and whole grains help maintain proper motility, allowing food to move through in a timely manner to produce a stool in a form and consistency with enough water to efficiently eliminate wastes, yet allow you to absorb the nutrients you need.

Resistant starches, ideally, also ferment in the large intestine, providing food for colonic organisms to make short-chain fatty acids and so on—a good thing! But again, you don't want too many gut flora eating fermentable foods in the small intestine. Their place to dine is in the next room down, but this shift in location of flora can change the entire dynamic of the gut and potentially your immune system and health.

Obese people with metabolic syndrome, who eat too much sugar and refined carbohydrates and too little good fiber, may have the wrong organisms camped out, not only causing gut trouble, but also actually helping them to gain weight, literally shifting their energy production. This topic opens a whole new world in medicine, associating obesity with those orchestra players in our gut, our microbiome.

## How Much Is "Regular"?

Although mainstream medicine may tell you that how many times a day you visit the porcelain throne—whether it's every two days, every four days, or three times a day—if it's what's always been your pattern, then it's normal for you. I beg to disagree. Just because it's what's always been doesn't mean it's what should be.

Understanding the role of elimination, gut motility and permeability, and nutrient adequacy, this antiquated guideline becomes poor advice. Although each of us has our own unique elimination patterns, our gut very much appreciates paying at least one bath-room trip a day to make a deposit. Two or more may be okay, too, depending on how much you eat and the form of the deposit.

Your gut flora, medications such as acid blockers, nutrient ad-equacy (particularly of magnesium), diet, fluid intake, and activ-ity level all affect your gut motility and the frequency and type of contribution you make to your bathroom visits. What goes in must come out, but *exactly what* goes in also determines what comes out. When it comes to the gut flora, food, especially carbohydrates, can affect the type and number of organisms. Additionally, if the bugs in the large intestine invite themselves up into the small intestines, they may overindulge. These changes in organisms can really dis-rupt the applecart—including changing the motility, initiating an inflammatory response, and increasing the mucosal permeability. Surgery, stress, the use of antibiotics, acne drugs, and other medi-cations, particularly acid-lowering drugs—all may change the bal-ance of these beneficial creatures. Acid blockers also can deplete key nutrients, particularly magnesium, that are helpful for gut motility.

For the gut to do its job well, it appreciates things to be a cer-tain way: periods of rest between eating, adequate fluids, chewing for the optimal signaling of hormones, enzymes to help break food down, and of course, the right diet. Elimination is a big part of how we detoxify our bodies, so regular but not too regular bathroom trips are essential to health.

## Key Takeaways

1. All carbohydrates are the primary fuel in our diet for gut organisms.
2. Ideally, fiber should have a positive role on the gut; however, gut-specific organisms and their location may influence how your body responds to fiber.
3. Prebiotics are fermentable carbohydrates that help stimulate growth of organisms, ideally in the large intestine.
4. A daily, formed bowel movement is a good goal for everyone—it's part of how we get rid of toxins. Optimizing gut flora and nutrients, such as magnesium, and determining the right carbohydrates, fiber, fluids, and activity level can make this happen.

# Part 4

## Determine How Carbohydrates Affect Your Body

# What Carb Camp Do You Fall Under?

# 20

# Determine Your Heart/Pancreas Carb Tolerance

Let's determine your carbohydrate tolerance—that is, how many carbohydrates your heart and pancreas can handle, as well as the amount that keeps your gut happy. Which path do you follow, or perhaps your paths cross? One body system may complain more than the other, but regardless, helping out one will help out the other.

To better determine your heart and pancreas tolerance to carbohydrates means answering a few questions about your medical history. Some of these questions may require a review with your physician.

1. *What are your blood sugar, hemoglobin A1C, and insulin levels?* If you consistently have any fasting blood sugars above 100 mg/dl, or random blood sugar above 140 mg/dl or a hemoglobin A1C equal to or above 5.7 percent, reducing carbohydrates should be in your future.

2. *What are your weight, body fat, and waist circumference?* A waist circumference greater than thirty-five inches for women and forty inches for men means too much visceral fat, the kind that raises your risk for insulin trouble. It is the most risky fat to store but is also the most receptive to exercise and carbohydrate reduction. If you have visceral fat on your belly, chances are that you are secreting more insulin to handle your carbohydrates than a lean person of equal height and weight. This is the easiest marker on which you can keep tabs.

3. *Do you have other risk factors*: high blood pressure (greater than 120/80 mm Hg), high triglycerides (greater than 150 mg/dL),

or low HDLs (less than 40 mg/dL)? Ask your physician to perform the more advanced lipid/cholesterol tests that reveal what kind of LDL and HDL cholesterol you have, including the lipoprotein: Lp(a). Knowing just the total number of cholesterol is obsolete, unless your total number is really high. Knowing the particle breakdown and the amount of oxidized LDL helps prevent overtreatment of high cholesterol with risky medications.

3. *What is your sensitive C-reactive protein (CRP)?* Sensitive CRP is an inflammatory marker. Levels above 3 mg/L may be a higher risk for metabolic syndrome and cardiac inflammation. Levels between 1 and 3 mg/L present an average risk, and less than 1 mg/L is a low risk.

4. *Do you have elevated liver enzymes?* Typically, measuring liver enzymes is part of a yearly physical. Ask your doctor if yours are normal. Alanine transaminase (ALT) and aspartate transaminase (AST) are the two enzymes most tested. Many factors may elevate these enzymes but it could indicate trouble with carbohydrate metabolism and or excess blood triglycerides. The good thing about the liver is that it can repair itself. Decreasing carbohydrates can reduce these enzymes back to normal.

5. *Do you have periodontal disease (gum disease)?* If you have chronic excessive bleeding in your mouth from inflamed gums, you may be at higher risk for heart disease. Excessive refined carbohydrates not only encourage more organisms to camp out in your mouth that can damage your teeth and gums but they also elevate your blood sugar, creating a systemic inflammatory state that does not help healing.

If you have any of the above risk factors your epigenetics and lifestyle may put you at risk for carbohydrate intolerance, entering metabolic syndrome territory. You may be susceptible to carbohydrates poorly affecting your blood sugar and insulin levels—the condition I refer to as *carbobesity*. Even if you have just one or two, you are at a metabolic crossroads and need to tread cautiously. Knowing that you possess these risk factors will help you understand the reason that you need to lower your carbohydrates.

## Key Takeaways

1. Determine your heart and pancreas carbohydrate tolerance by looking at some key markers in your medical history.
2. Any of these markers may suggest you need to lower or change your intake of carbohydrates.
3. Review these markers with your physician.

# 21

# How to Determine Your Gut Carbohydrate Tolerance

The type of carbohydrate you eat, the location of any gut distur-bance, and how often you visit the bathroom contribute to and reflect your gut carbohydrate tolerance. Additionally, the lifestyle you lead—including exercise, medications, illnesses, surgeries, and stress—influence your ability to digest carbohydrates.

The first step in understanding your gut carbohydrate tolerance is to determine if you have any other major GI condition.

I'm thinking primarily of cancers, ulcerative colitis, Crohn's disease and celiac disease, and other conditions such as gastropare-sis. This may require some testing from your physician. Be cautious of overtesting, but at least a celiac blood test is prudent for most adults, especially if you have GI symptoms. Also, consider a regu-lar recommended colonoscopy. A bird's-eye view can help rule out some of these bigger-ticket items.

## Celiac and Gluten Testing: What's the Difference?

Celiac and gluten sensitivity testing are varied and can be con-fusing but may be helpful to give forewarning of your body's toler-ance to gluten. Tests include measuring gut villi damage, but these don't directly determine gluten sensitivity.

### Total IgA

IgA is an antibody or immunoglobulin, one of a variety of an-tibodies in our bodies' arsenals to defend ourselves. IgA is most prevalent in the GI tract. Perhaps the most frequent misstep in celiac testing is not measuring the total amount of IgA. It is imperative that, along with any other test that measures IgA, a total IgA must be taken, too. This helps ensure that you produce enough IgA to muster up a reliable response to the other tests. Up to 10 percent of people with celiac disease are IgA deficient, and 3 to 5 percent of the general population are IgA deficient. Without a total IgA measurement, the other IgA measurements are unreliable.

IgG is another immunoglobin that we produce, not as prevalent in the gut, but still used to diagnose celiac disease and gut sensitivities, especially if IgA is deficient.

## *tTG IgA, IgG*

Tissue transglutaminase is a specific antibody made to fight tissue damage in the small intestine. It is a sensitive indicator of damage from gluten in celiac disease. It is the more common blood test used to diagnosis celiac disease.

## *EMA IgA, IgG*

Endomesial antibodies IgA is an older marker but still somewhat reliable in detecting damage from gluten and the presence of celiac disease and is often used if other results are questionable.

## *Anti-DGP-Deanimated Gliadin Peptide*

This is a newer test and measures an immune response to a specific fragment of the gluten molecule. DGP is becoming more reliable than EMA or tTG to detect gut damage and celiac disease. More celiac centers in the United States are using this marker, especially if IgA is deficient.

# Nonceliac Gluten Sensitivity or Intolerance

The medical community is paying more attention to this condition, and studies are under way trying to identity more specific biomarkers. Essentially, it is a sensitivity to gluten that produces an immune response but is not celiac disease.

For now, the most accepted way to detect nonceliac gluten sensitivity is by clinical symptoms and the older celiac tests. These tests measure a response to gliadin, one of the proteins in gluten. The tests were formerly used to diagnosis celiac disease but are not accurate to measure actual gut damage; a positive response is noteworthy information.

Their drawback is that some people with nonceliac sensitivity don't test positive for antigliadin antibodies; however, they may test positive for fecal IgA antibodies. Fecal antibody testing has not yet gained mainstream acceptance. Although some labs do fecal testing, insurance does not cover it.

The following tests may help you identify a sensitivity to gluten that is not celiac disease.

- Antigliadin antibody IgA (IgA-gliadin antibody)
- Antigliadin antibody IgG (IgG-gliadin antibody)
- Fecal IgA antibodies
- Fecal anti-tTG IgA antibodies

## Gene Testing for Celiac Disease

It is believed that about 97 percent of people who have celiac disease have the HLA DQ2 and HLA DQ8 genes. Knowing if you have the potential to develop celiac disease may help you avoid it, but you can have the gene and never develop celiac disease. Also, 50 percent of type 1 diabetes patients have the same HLA gene.

Other testing may include imaging via endoscopy or colonoscopy. Officially, the medical community requires biopsy from an endoscopy and blood test for a positive celiac disease diagnosis. Also, keep in mind that other things cause villous damage in the small intestine, including NSAIDs such as aspirin, ibuprofen, and naproxen. Officially, then, a celiac disease diagnosis requires both blood testing and an endoscopy.

## Testing for IBS (Irritable Bowel Syndrome) and SIBO (Small Intestine Bacterial Overgrowth)

IBS is a functional GI disorder. The diagnosis is often given after other conditions have been ruled out. IBS is a complex condition probably involving gut dysbiosis, gut hyperpermeability, inflammation, hypersensitivity, and alteration of gut neurotransmitters.

SIBO is an overgrowth of organisms that are normally not present in the small intestine. It can create excessive bloating, gas, and discomfort from the organisms "eating" certain carbohydrates as they pass through. It may also change the mucosal permeability. SIBO occurs in up to 70 to 80 percent of people with irritable bowel syndrome.

## *Lactulose/Glucose Breath Tests*

A lactulose/glucose breath test is not conclusive but is a start for those who want more proof of SIBO. The sugar lactulose or sometimes glucose is administered orally, and then a clinician measures the amount and type of gases breathed out. These gases are a by-product of the organisms in your small intestine eating the carbs that you provide. Differences in hydrogen, methane, and hydrogen sulfide gases reflect the type of gut organisms and also are associated with patterns of constipation and diarrhea.

## *Hydrochloric acid (HCL) Testing*

The Heidelberg test is the more formal, medically approved way to measure HCL adequacy of your stomach. Low HCL puts you at risk for SIBO and a few other GI disorders. How the test works is you swallow a small, encapsulated radio transmitter, which measures the pH of the stomach at rest as well as after administering baking soda, which is quite alkaline. The Heidelberg test is expensive and not performed often by physicians. A close second for effectiveness, however, is a home test that involves taking a supplement of HCL, called betaine HCL. There are a number of brands and ultimately if you need to supplement use a brand that also contains pepsin. Although the home test is generally quite safe for most people and correcting a low level can give you tremendous health benefits, please heed this red tape warning. It is not risk free and consider doing under the supervision of a physician or clinician familiar with its administration. Also, it is not a one-size-fits-all test. As with most things with the body, your results may vary from your neighbors.

Caution: Do not use this home HCL test if you have peptic ulcer disease or are regularly consuming any anti-inflammatory medicines such as corticosteroids, aspirin, ibuprofen, or other NSAIDs. These medications can damage the stomach lining, so further irritation may increase your risk for bleeding. Also do not empty the HCL capsules into beverages because direct contact on tissues or teeth can be corrosive. The stomach is designed to handle the acid, but most of the rest of your body is not.

---

### Home self-test for stomach HCL adequacy

1. Take one 350–750 mg capsule of betaine HCL with a protein-containing meal, preferably at least 15 grams (two ounces of meat, chicken, or fish). A normal response for a person with adequate HCL is a heartburn-type burning sensation. Makes sense, right? If you are making enough HCL, then you don't need more. If you feel no pain or discomfort, then chances are you are making less. To confirm your suspicions, repeat this dosage of one pill for two more meals with protein.

2. On the second day, if you still feel no pain, increase your dosage to two pills per protein-containing meal. Continue to increase by one pill every two days up until eight capsules per meal at a time. You will know if you've taken too much by a burning, heartburn sensation.

3. When you've identified the number of pills that causes discomfort, cut back by one pill. For example, if five pills give you a burning sensation, then four pills may be your proper dosage. Smaller meals with less protein may require fewer pills.

---

If you do experience heartburn discomfort, you can neutralize the acid with ½–1 teaspoon of baking soda in a cup of water or milk. If you continue to experience discomfort, contact your doctor. The number of pills may seem like a lot, but a normal, healthy human stomach makes much more HCL. The goal is to guide your stomach back to making the right levels, and there are ways to help it along, including using apple cider vinegar, digestive bitters, and deglycerized licorice. Work with a physician or clinician who can help you determine what dosage is best for you and the need for further supplements.

## Endotoxin/Lipopolysaccharide Testing

This type of testing is on the horizon; some labs provide it now. Lipopolysaccharides (LPS) are found on the cell surface of certain bacteria. When too much of the wrong bacteria hangs out in the gut, it can form a biofilm, or very strong bond to the mucosal wall. It may trigger inflammation and begin the process of immune dysregulation. A marker for these biofilms may be measuring lipopolysaccharides.

## Urinary Organic Acids and Stool Profiles

The organisms in our gut release byproducts from their metabolizing and feasting on the food we provide them. These byproducts show up in the urine and high levels of some may provide markers for people with certain gastrointestinal or neurological symptoms. Some of the elevated acids that are associated with microbial overgrowth include benzoate, hippurate, cresol, and phenylacetate. Medicine has traditionally only tested for certain organic acid markers when testing for genetic inborn errors of metabolism in newborns. But we are learning that these acids may be markers for measuring gut dysbiosis that can be treated with a change in diet and supplementation.

Stool testing can be revealing too, but keep in mind probably does not show what's going on in the small intestine, but rather more what's happening in the colon. Its value is controversial in GI circles; however, it can help diagnosis parasites and other organisms that just shouldn't be there. It can also show how many of those beneficial fatty acids you make as well as if your stools contain too much fat, a marker for malabsorption.

* * *

## Other Clues Associated with Gut-Carbohydrate Tolerance

**Other autoimmune diseases.** People with autoimmune diseases—including type 1 diabetes, celiac disease, thyroid disorders such as Hashimoto's thyroiditis and Graves' disease, and multiple sclerosis—may have a higher risk of gut permeability.

**Zonulin levels.** Zonulin is a protein whose levels correspond to greater intestinal permeability. People with type 1 diabetes and celiac disease have higher zonulin levels and greater intestinal permeability. One study has shown that people with glucose intolerance and obesity produced more zonulin, a possible association between the gut and insulin resistance.

**Bowel patterns.** Constipation and diarrhea reflect gut motility and permeability, influenced by the flora and what you eat. Keep track of your bowel patterns and notice any associations with certain foods.

**Belching, bloating, acid reflux, and excessive flatulence.** Belching and acid reflux are common when the wrong organisms start to multiply, particularly if you are taking an acid blocker. Difficult-to-digest proteins such as gluten and sugars such as fructose or lactose may also be associated with bloating and acid reflux. Flatuence or "passing gas" is normal and healthy; however, excessive flatulence may be an indication of excessive organisms in the wrong places.

**GI cramping or abdominal pain**. Pain is always a marker to heed. It may reflect inflammation, obstruction, infection, or bleeding. Don't let pain become chronic without checking with a physician.

**Caution:** Although adjusting your intake of carbohydrates may help some or all of these conditions, be careful not to self-diagnose. Prolonged bleeding, diarrhea, constipation, or pain requires a medical checkup.

## Key Takeaways

1. Checking your GI carbohydrate tolerance requires ruling out certain other major GI conditions. Adjusting your carbohydrates may help all of them.

2. Consider a celiac blood test if you have any GI symptoms for longer than six months. Celiac can present with many other symptoms unrelated to the GI tract.

3. IBS is a complex condition, usually determined after other GI conditions have been ruled out. SIBO may be present in IBS and many other GI conditions. A breath test may help with diagnosis.

4. Checking other signs and symptoms can also help manage your carbohydrate tolerance. Be careful not to self-diagnose. Pain, fever, and bleeding are important markers to address with a physician.

# 22

# A Word about Celiac Disease and Zonulin

I've been attending celiac disease conferences for over twenty years, and perhaps the most impressive piece of information I've learned is that no one celiac-afflicted person looks like another. Yes, there are common themes, and certainly GI complaints may be part of them, but not all. A person with undiagnosed celiac disease can be obese, thin, or muscular; have no GI complaints or lots of them; have fatigue or anemia, and the list goes on. I have seen patients that fit all of these descriptions. My practice includes many who were diagnosed later in life and look back in their life and say, "Okay, so that's why!"

Without question, anyone who has any GI symptoms for longer than six months should be tested for celiac disease or gluten sensitivity. Currently gluten must be present in the diet for accurate results, so the very thing that causes the damage cannot be removed to diagnosis the disease accurately. I believe that many people who are not officially diagnosed begin eating gluten-free to "heal" themselves, which may be okay; however, an official diagnosis may also get you insurance benefits, as well as more invested care.

A diagnosis of celiac disease is not perfect. Most American physicians use endoscopy and the total IgA and tTG blood tests, which actually show later stages of celiac disease when villi damage has already occurred. Where are the people in the beginning stages of celiac disease? Those intestinal microvilli—fingerlike projections that absorb nutrients—don't become damaged and flatten overnight. Research shows that partial damage may not show up in blood tests. Are we missing a stage of celiac disease? Also, the results of the blood test don't always predict the results of the endoscopy. Newer celiac disease blood tests are being developed—but are not available yet for the public—that allow testing without the need to eat gluten.

You may be celiac-negative at age thirty and then celiac-positive at forty. Or perhaps you had celiac issues all along but did not have enough damage to test positive. Maybe your immune system and the microflora in your gut protected you until you had a life change: pregnancy, antibiotics, long-term antacid use. Changes in your gut organisms may change your protection. I don't know the answer, but I wonder if people who carry the celiac disease gene could perhaps be better protected by avoiding gluten or decreasing their gluten load or eating an optimal combination of carbohydrates that fosters better gut flora, which may help them build the right immunity to handle the gluten that they do eat so they don't ever become celiac-positive.

People with celiac disease must completely avoid gluten, including sources such as Communion wafers and shared toasters or cutting boards. Even cross-contamination can keep antibody levels elevated. People with celiac disease have greater health risks, especially if undiagnosed, including a higher risk for lymphoma.

## Zonulin

Celiac disease is all about intestinal permeability and has dramatically increased medicine's learning curve on this subject. Intestinal permeability is why celiac disease is related to other autoimmune diseases such as Hashimoto's thyroiditis, Graves' disease, and rheumatoid arthritis.

Now I want to briefly introduce you to zonulin, a protein marker for measuring mucosal permeability that we all produce. With celiac disease, zonulin is significantly elevated, increasing the intestinal mucosal wall's permeability. It makes those tight junction gatekeepers in the mucosal wall that specifically open for certain molecules open even wider. Zonulin has helped confirm that excess intestinal permeability or leaky gut exists. Gliadin, the protein in gluten, is believed to be the provoking factor for increasing gut permeability in celiac disease, but the jury is still out if other factors may play a role.

Since we all produce zonulin, some researchers believe that even with nonceliac gluten intolerance, when we eat gluten, the permeability of our intestinal wall opens more than normal but then closes quickly and our immune system handles it at that time. But with too heavy a gluten load or with health changes, your immune system may no longer handle it, giving gluten a potentially pivotal role in transforming the progression of disease.

Certain bacteria increase zonulin levels, too. Our small intestine may try to protect itself by recognizing certain organisms as dangerous, so we make zonulin to open the door and let them out—but at a price if those tight junctions don't return to optimal permeability. Vibrio, the organism in cholera, is one example in which zonulin levels are higher.

Increased zonulin levels and increased intestinal permeability are also present in type 1 diabetes, an autoimmune disease that attacks the beta cells of the pancreas. Most recently a Spanish study has shown a relationship between insulin resistance, obesity, and zonulin levels. Obese subjects with insulin resistance had significantly higher zonulin levels than subjects without insulin resistance, further connecting the roles of gut wall permeability, gut bacteria, and insulin dysregulation.

## Key Takeaways

1. Celiac disease is a condition in which gluten—the protein in wheat, barley, and rye—cannot be digested or absorbed. It can present with a number of symptoms. Don't hesitate to ask your physician for a blood test, especially if you've had GI symptoms for more than six months.
2. Zonulin is a protein in our blood that controls how the tight junction gates in the mucosal wall of the small intestine open. Research shows that a variety of factors may risk these gates to open and not close as readily, including gluten, diabetes, and a number of organisms. Zonulin levels may become a marker to assess gut health and immunity.

# 23

# The Gluten-Free Train, FODMAPs, and Other Stuff

Not everyone is on board the gluten-free train, but the research shows well enough to me that gluten is a tough protein in food to digest, especially as we age and especially if you have other risk factors. When we think of protein, we don't typically think of gluten. We think of other amino acids that are in meat, chicken and fish. But gluten is an amino acid found in wheat, barley, and rye, and it can get through the mucosal wall intact fairly easily, instead of being broken down into smaller fragments, leaving this larger protein in your blood for your body to decide what to do.

Thanks to decades of cross-mutations, the wheat in our food supply now may be different from the wheat in the food supply fifty years ago, a hundred years ago, and from biblical times, which potentially makes the gluten different as well. Plus, gluten is just more prevalent in the diet. Think about how often your gut encounters gluten found in wheat, barley, and rye, plus added ingredients in processed foods. Although the research is limited, cosmetics and beauty products may also affect those who are gluten sensitive.

If you eat bagels, bread, pretzels, crackers, pasta, cereals, condiments, and so on, you are eating gluten from up to ten or more different sources per day. When it comes to restricting gluten, I don't believe you are losing many nutrients. I can't lose sleep over taking out some or even all of the grains from the diet if necessary to help someone feel better and be healthier, which forms much of the basis for my rationale in determining which foods to restrict. I go back to my fundamentals in nutrition and strive to consume the most nutrient-dense foods, meaning the foods with the most vitamins, minerals, phytochemicals, and fiber. Most gluten-containing foods are refined carbohydrates, raising your blood sugar and requiring insulin. Even whole-grain wheat raises your blood sugar as much as white wheat.

Although bread and wheat may have great philosophical, religious, and emotional value for people, that doesn't mean it is healthy for us to eat the quantities we eat today. We rely on and are emotionally attached to gluten and the foods that contain it. Most whole grains do not contain enough nutrients to justify keeping them—or at least a lot of them if you are at risk for metabolic syndrome or gut dysbiosis. You can get what few nutrients they offer (B vitamins and fiber) elsewhere, certainly at least temporarily while you try a gluten-free lifestyle.

Tread carefully, or better yet, walk away from most gluten-free foods that are not naturally gluten-free. For example, yogurt is naturally gluten-free. But cookies or bread that once were made with wheat but then use gluten-free grains as substitutes are not. The grains and ingredients used to replace gluten-containing grains include tapioca starch, potato starch, and others—and, of course, lots of sugar, all raising your blood sugar and providing minimal nutrients. We discuss these foods more later, but many gluten-free products are still a ticket to more processed, refined carbohydrates.

## FODMAPs

FODMAPs are rapidly becoming well-known in belly circles. It is an acronym for a group of fermentable sugars that can be difficult to digest (fermentable oligosaccharides, disaccharides, monosaccharides, and polyols). These sugars include fructose, lactose, fructans, galactans, and polyols and are found in many healthy foods, particularly dairy, fruits, and vegetables.

We all have the enzymes to digest the sugars lactose and fructose. True lactase deficiency is a rare condition. However, lactase deficiency as a result of a compromising gut problem is not rare. Likely, if you have any gut wall damage, then you have fewer enzymes for lactose and fructose, and these two sugars may be partially undigested, leaving them to be fermented in the small intestine and providing a nice meal for organisms.

The high fructose corn syrup found in many foods adds to our fructose load, which many guts cannot handle. Fructose malabsorption, unrelated to hereditary fructose malabsorption (HFI), is becoming more common. Fruits containing higher fructose include apples, pears, and mangoes. Honey and agave are sweeteners that are also high in fructose.

For the sugars in foods such as fructans and galactans, humans do not possess the enzymes to digest them. Fructans are found primarily in wheat and fruit but also onions and garlic, and galactans are found primarily in legumes.

Restricting most FODMAPs foods indefinitely is not recommended since they are found in many nutrient-dense foods, especially fruits and vegetables. Many people with IBS and celiac disease are sensitive to FODMAPs foods and benefit from restricting them temporarily. Although I fully recognize the benefits of restricting FODMAPs in helping heal a sensitive gut, I prefer to restrict some less nutrient-dense foods first and move on to certain FODMAPs later. Some less nutrient-dense foods contain high FODMAPs sugars, too—all the more reason to cut them out, for example, the fructans in bread.

Guidelines for restricting FODMAPs aim to reduce the total amount per sitting to 0.5 grams, while also maintaining limits on each FODMAPs group. Each group has a tolerable limit based on research of people with IBS and SIBO consuming these foods. Limiting FODMAPs and reintroducing foods can be restrictive and confusing but have beneficial effects when accomplished with a dietitian or nutritionist who understands the approach.

Monash University in Australia has been the pioneer in FODMAPs and IBS research. Its website, http://www.med.monash.edu/cecs/gastro/fodmap/, offers a wealth of tips and information.

## Is It Gluten or Fructans?

Removing gluten in wheat gives you a double benefit. You're removing a high-insulin-demand food, and you are also reducing your intake of fructans, a FODMAPs sugar, not to be confused with fructose. Even the healthiest of guts over time and with age may easily have trouble with fructans, the sugar in wheat. By removing gluten you have removed two potential irritants. It's nearly impossible to differentiate whether fructans or gluten bothers your gut, since they are in similar foods, and if you have any negative gut permeability, you may be sensitive to both.

## Gluten vs FODMAPs

An important concept to keep in mind is that comparing FODMAPs and gluten is like comparing "apples and oranges" or shall I say apples and chicken. FODMAPs are sugars and gluten is a protein, which means it contains amino acids. The confusing issue is that gluten is a protein that happens to be in foods that contain high levels of carbohydrates or sugars. They are structurally different and behave in the body differently.

FODMAPs' potential negative effect on the gut stems from their creating an imbalance of organisms, which may then cause an inflammatory response. Proteins typically are what the body may interpret as foreign and respond by making an antibody. So, gluten's potential effect on our body is from the inability to break it down and it ending up in our blood as a less digested protein, leaving our immune system deciding what to do. Medicine is just beginning to study these components of foods and their associations with various symptoms and conditions, but their pathway to creating inflammation and an immune response may be different, which may determine the best practices for treatment.

## Gastroparesis

*Gastroparesis*, a condition in which stomach emptying is delayed, can result from a variety of reasons but most commonly is associated with diabetes. Any backup in the GI track is not good, so one occurring this high up just sets the scene for further imbalance. Interestingly, gastroperesis is associated with SIBO, perhaps because food stays too long in the stomach and encourages organisms to travel upward. No one knows for sure. But an excess of carbohydrates elevates blood sugars, leading to diabetes, and diabetes can lead to gastroparesis.

## Key Takeaways

1. Gluten is a difficult protein in foods to digest and may be problematic not only for people with celiac disease.

2. Many foods with gluten are refined grains that raise blood sugar and may cause GI distress.

3. FODMAPs are sugars found in a variety of foods that may be difficult to digest and create an imbalance of organisms, especially for people with IBS and other GI conditions. Reducing the total amount of FODMAPs can help improve a sensitive gut.

# 24

# Carbs and Fiber: How Low Do You Go?

When we eat certain fibers found in whole plant foods like apples, the good bacteria in our large intestine ferment them into short-chain fatty acids (SCFA) like butyrate, propionate, and acetate. Butyrate receives the most attention, and researchers believe it may have anti-inflammatory effects, help the immune response, increase insulin sensitivity, and may be even be helpful in the treatment of diseases of the colon such as Crohn's, IBS, ulcerative colitis, and colon cancer. The optimal level of butyrate acids for colon health is undetermined, but we know we like them; their presence is beneficial.

FODMAPs research has contributed a great deal to understanding which carbohydrates are more fermentable, although we are still learning the differences between many types of sugars, starches, and fibers. We're also learning the differences with which fibers increase short-chain fatty acid production. Older studies have shown that insoluble fibers increase butyrate, but more recent data show that so do certain soluble fibers and some resistant starches as well.

Generally speaking, the more fermentable fiber consumed particularly as fruits and vegetables, potentially the more short-chain fatty acids produced. One of the risks of long-term very low-carbohydrate (VLC) diets is the potentially harmful effects they may have on reducing beneficial gut flora. Essentially they may starve both the good and bad bugs, much like how most antibiotics kill both good and bad bacteria.

In the *short term*, less than 50 grams of carbohydrates a day (a VLC diet) may be therapeutic for gut infections by giving all organisms less to eat and can have a profound positive effect on insulin resistance and weight control. But if practiced for too long, a VLC diet can be risky to the gut. The goal is competition—more of the good than the bad, as well as a diversity of organisms. Given that people today are exposed to many more carcinogens and environmental triggers than thousands of years ago, we may need as strong a weaponry as we can muster to protect ourselves. Our bodies may need the strongest gut flora now more than ever, which may mean finding the right type and amount of fiber to suit your body.

*Back to that million-dollar question:* How many carbohydrates are necessary to obtain the health benefits from the healthy organisms in the colon before those carbs promote excess blood sugar and insulin production? We know that some people are so metabolically resistant that ketosis is a beneficial option. But we must keep in mind the benefits to the colon and potential immune modulation that may occur from eating a certain amount of fermentable carbohydrates. Again, my hope is that most people could find a carbohydrate balance that is low enough to keep blood sugars and insulin healthy, while high enough and with the right type to maintain a healthy gut too. Perhaps one leads to the other.

## Key Takeaways

1. Fewer than 50 grams a day of carbohydrates (a VLC diet) may dramatically improve insulin resistance and weight loss, and decrease heart disease risk.
2. Long-term VLC intake of fewer than 50 grams a day may risk inadequate fiber and nutrients from fruits and vegetables and other fermentable carbohydrates that may have benefits for the large intestine.
3. How many carbohydrates are necessary to reduce blood sugar and insulin levels, while also maintaining optimal colonic organisms, is probably an individual matter and needs more research.

# Part 5

## How to Adjust the Carbs in Your Diet

# Two Approaches

You may be more insulin-resistant-dominant or GI-symptom-dominant; you could even be both. Regardless, reducing the total quantity of carbohydrates will help. If you are GI dominant, the type of carbohydrates will be important, too. The type of carbohydrates may also have an impact on insulin tolerance—higher in fiber helping insulin resistance.

This part of the book presents two systematic approaches to reducing carbohydrates. One reduces by counting grams and the other by reducing carbohydrates in layers. With both of these approaches, adequate protein and healthy, unprocessed fats should make up the rest of your calories. For the best bang for your protein buck, aim to include 1 to 5 ounces of protein at all meals, depending on your protein requirement. This approach allows for the best satiety value and the best use of amino acids.

Also, a lower-carbohydrates diet usually results in a higher-fat diet, which doesn't give you permission to drink from the oil bottle or throw caution to the wind with total calories consumed. But depending on how much you lower your carbohydrates, you will have more room for a variety of healthy fats. Because fat does not stimulate insulin, and if the fats are healthy fats, research shows that your risk of heart disease will go down, not up. Remember, excessive carbohydrates drive the elevated blood sugars, and high triglyceride levels that increase inflammation and cardiac risk.

*Any lowering of carbohydrates is going to help lower insulin demand.* It gets tricky, however, in knowing how to adjust the type of carbohydrates to treat GI symptoms, since some people are sensitive to FODMAPs, some more to starch, or some just to gluten . . . but manipulating the type may well help your belly.

# 25

# Counting Carbs

Reducing carbohydrates by counting grams allows you to know exactly where you stand with quantity. This approach involves more work in the beginning, but you gain some lifelong knowledge of how to balance your diet. Lowering carb intake also has a high success rate in improving insulin resistance, as shown by Eric Westman's low-carbohydrate program at Duke University.

Reducing carbohydrates by counting grams can also be used for GI intolerances, but as you count grams, pay attention to the type of carbohydrates you eat.

To reduce carbohydrates by counting grams, let's first look at different carbohydrate zones and get an idea of what people normally eat. No medically agreed-upon requirement for carbohydrates exists. Keep in mind, historically, the American Diabetes Association and the Academy of Nutrition and Dietetics have not recommended that people eat a diet with fewer than 40 percent of calories coming from carbohydrate. The United States Department of Agriculture's My Plate website states that, "calories matter when it comes to body weight, not the calorie source." My experience and research challenges this statement. Research shows benefits for some individuals at VLC levels, and we know the damage that can occur at very high levels above 300 grams of carbohydrates per day. Consider the accompanying box, which shows varying ranges of carbohydrate consumption with their potential risks and benefits. No one range is best for everyone.

## Carbohydrates to Fit Your Tolerance Zones

**Greater than 300 grams per day.** Most endurance athletes and traditional sports nutrition guidelines encourage even up to **500 to 600 grams a day** or 1 to 4 grams per kilogram of body weight, depending on length of exercise. Recommendations are based on athletic performance, glycogen storage, and glucose utilization as a fuel source. Research does not, however, consider the long-term demand for insulin on the pancreas.

**250–350 grams per day.** Typical American diet, and although your genes may have an influence here, this amount is usually too much to allow weight loss in most people over forty years of age, except with increased exercise.

**250 grams per day.** As shown in the traditional food pyramid guidelines, this amount of carbohydrate constitutes approximately 50 percent of the calories in a 2,000-calorie diet. If you have high blood sugar, insulin resistance, or trouble losing weight, this may be too many carbohydrates for you.

**200–250 grams per day.** This is 40 to 50 percent of the calories in a 2,000-calorie diet and is the lowest amount of carbohydrate that the American Diabetes Association and Academy of Nutrition and Dietetics officially recommend for carbohydrate consumption, according to the My Plate guidelines for a healthy diet. Many type 1 diabetics have difficulty managing medications with this amount of carbohydrates, and most type 2 diabetics have difficulty with preventing weight gain, especially without exercise. But it is a start for eating fewer carbohydrates.

**130–200 grams per day.** Not considered low carbohydrate by medical standards but lower than what many people eat. Some but not all people may notice weight loss or at least weight maintenance, but usually that requires consistent, dedicated exercise.

**Less than 130 grams per day.** Considered low carbohydrate by medical standards; you will see weight loss, improvement in insulin resistance, and improvement in gut sensitivities at this level of carbohydrates, particularly if you pay attention to the type.

**75–130 grams per day.** Potential sweet zone for weight loss or weight maintenance, with improvement in insulin resistance without going into ketosis. Particular attention must be given to selecting your best carbohydrates and fats with varied fruits and vegetables.

**50–100 grams a day.** Weight loss made much easier; possible ketosis for some. Extra attention must be made to select your best carbohydrates and fats with varied fruits and vegetables.

**25–50 grams a day.** Ketosis and fast weight loss can occur here, though such levels are hard, but possible, to maintain. Requires prolonged restriction of grains, as well as many fruits and starchy vegetables, though small amounts of selected fruits and vegetables are allowed. Risk of inadequate fiber and loss of their benefits.

**0–25 grams a day.** Ketosis and fast weight loss and improvement of seizures for certain epileptics. Difficult to maintain long term, and risk of inadequate fiber and loss of their associated benefits.

## Start Counting

To start counting grams of carbohydrates, become familiar with food labels, as well as the carbohydrate servings for food groups. Best to spread your carbohydrates out throughout the day to help lessen the load on your pancreas and gut at any one sitting. Be sure to ingest adequate protein and adequate essential fats. The glycemic index comes in handy, too, where low-glycemic-index foods should make up the bulk of your carbohydrates. Although we're not counting calories, it doesn't mean you can throw caution to the wind with limitless calories.

If your diet was excessively high in calories and carbohydrates to start, reducing both calories and carbohydrates will help. Generally, with fewer carbohydrates, particularly if under 130 grams a day, in order for that plan to be sustainable, fat intake should modestly increase. Ketosis requires a more dramatic increase in fat in order to maintain the ketosis because so few calories are coming from carbohydrates. But regardless of ketosis, because a higher amount of your calories are from fat and with adequate protein, your appetite is easier to manage.

Depending on how many carbohydrates you decide to try, aim to distribute those carbs fairly evenly in two to three meals and snacks. For example, if your want to eat 130 grams per day, aim for 30 to 40 grams of carbohydrates per meal and 0 to 10 grams per snack. You may need to go lower, or you may be able to go higher. Refer back to chapter 7 of this book titled, "How Much Lives Where" for the average carbohydrate content of various food groups. Remember, these numbers are really rough. Better to read your food label and see exactly the amount of carbohydrates listed for that food under "total carbohydrates." Also look closely at the serving size. As mentioned earlier, it's a rare, usually conscious effort to eat just one-third of a cup of cooked pasta or one-quarter of a large bagel.

Most processed low-fat foods contain higher amounts of carbohydrates. When manufacturers take out the fat, frequently they put back in some form of carbohydrates. Remember that it's okay to increase your fat intake as you lower carbohydrates. But aim for naturally occurring fats in foods such as nuts, seeds, avocados, butter, olive oil, coconut oil, cheese, and unsweetened full-fat dairy.

Check out the following Internet links for the carbohydrate content of foods:

- http://www.diabetes.org/food-and-fitness/food/what-can-i-eat/understanding-carbohydrates/carbohydrate-counting. html#sthash.ZKvapSte.dpuf
- www.calorieking.com
- http://www.nal.usda.gov

## Key Takeaways

1. Counting daily grams of carbohydrates is a good exercise for everyone. More than 300 grams per day without exercise leads to weight gain in most people.

2. Ketosis usually occurs with fewer than 50 grams of carbohydrates per day.

3. Any reduction in carbohydrates will help the pancreas. Daily carb intakes between 75 and 130 grams per day will promote weight loss and lower blood sugars and triglycerides—without going into ketosis.

4. Divide carbohydrates somewhat evenly over meals and snacks.

5. A lower-carb diet usually results in a higher-fat diet, depending on the level of carbohydrate reduction. Ketosis requires the greatest elevation of dietary fat. Dietary fat does not stimulate insulin.

# 26

# Layer by Layer:
# The Seven-Layered Carb Plan

To reduce carbohydrates in layers, one of my compasses initially for determining the amount and type is the overall nutrient density of the food. After that, change the carbohydrate choice to suit your symptoms following some of the points we discussed earlier about the high-risk components that some carbs—that is, gluten and FODMAPs—may present to the belly. Allow at least five days between removing individual foods or reintroducing a food to better determine the association of a food with certain symptoms. More than one exposure to a food may be necessary to accurately identify a food intolerance.

Also, it is usually not necessary to remove all seven layers to see health improvements but if you do, maintain the restriction for four to six weeks; then add back the most nutrient-dense foods one by one, with at least five days between each new food. Adding back FODMAPs requires a little more care, as some foods contain more than one FODMAPs.

This approach requires no counting of grams but reducing by food groups according to nutrient density. For many people it's enough to get you to a better place without being too restrictive or thinking about numbers. Some people like to ease themselves into changes; this approach is a good start.

So, which layer first?

**1. Simple, remove or reduce the foods that are high in sugar.** Limit the most obvious sources of sugars: sodas, candy, cookies, cakes, and pastries. All of these foods are high in carbohydrates and low in nutrients, offering the proverbial "empty calories." By reducing these foods you are likely lowering your carbohydrates by at least 75 grams a day, probably much more, depending on how much you eat. Just decreasing the carbohydrate load decreases your blood sugar as well as the demand on your pancreas for insulin.

See what happens, check your blood sugar, and watch for any weight changes. While you are doing this, keep all other sources of carbohydrates—fruits, vegetables, grains, and other starches—stable, but take away or significantly decrease sweets. This is an excellent start.

**2. Remove the gluten layer.** This is an initial, greater attempt to address GI symptoms and possibly other symptoms if you have nonceliac gluten sensitivity, but it can also help your blood sugar. Reduce servings of gluten without replacing them with a gluten-free processed substitute. Gluten-free replacement foods are made of high-glycemic-index carbohydrates, including potato starch, tapioca, soy, and rice. "High-glycemic-index" means that they raise your blood sugar quickly.

Although the glycemic index is not the only factor in determining how quickly carbohydrates raise your blood sugar, generally the more high-glycemic-index foods you eat, the more your pancreas has to work. Plus, these starches that replace gluten are no better nutritionally, except they are gluten-free, which primarily provides alternative foods for gluten-sensitive guts but also keeps their insulin load high. Truthfully, the most appropriate people for gluten-free substitutes are people with celiac disease or nonceliac sensitivities who need to gain weight, or people for whom weight is not an issue or who have normal blood sugars.

An exception to eating completely gluten-free for people without celiac disease is to include certain gluten-containing grains such as sprouted grains and Einkorn wheat. Sprouting is a stage that occurs as a seed grows into a fully mature grain. Remember, grains are seeds of grass; some research suggests that the sprouting stage may offer health benefits. Einkorn wheat is considered one of the first grains of many cultures, and some research suggests that its gluten may be easier to digest.

When you remove gluten from your diet, if you continue to eat gluten-free grains such as rice, quinoa, and potato, eat them in as close to their whole form as possible, not as an ingredient listing—whole potato vs. potato starch on a label, whole rice cooked vs. rice flour on a label, whole quinoa, whole oatmeal cooked, and so on.

*Goal: Aim for zero to two servings maximum per day.*

**3. Remove or reduce all grains (gasp!).** If you've stuck with removing the gluten layer, you've already removed bread and some of the emotionally tougher foods for people to omit. If you're still experiencing GI symptoms or your blood sugar is high, remove all other grains—including rice, corn, quinoa, millet, and oatmeal (see grains list)—or limit them to one to two servings per day; it's your choice where you keep them. All grains are concentrated sources of carbohydrates and raise blood sugars and provide food for a compromised gut.

*Note:* You can try to keep sourdough, spelt, or sprouted breads, which can be lower in fructans and gluten, depending on how they are made. Generally, sourdough rye breads are lower in fructans than sourdough wheat. If your blood sugar and weight are okay and you can be moderate, go for keeping them. Let your belly and blood sugars help you decide.

*Goal: Aim for zero to two servings per day maximum of any grain. Keep tuberous root vegetables such as potatoes and sweet potatoes (yams) in your diet. Continue to eat fruits, vegetables, nuts, seeds, and dairy.*

**4. Remove all remaining starchy vegetables: tuberous root and others.**

This layer can be done all together or by individual foods. Largely you are removing potatoes and peas, the remaining starchy vegetables.

*Goal: Zero to two servings of starchy vegetables per day.*

**5. Remove or reduce dairy, especially sweetened yogurts and dairy drinks.**

If you know you are lactose intolerant, then by all means reduce this layer sooner. I do not unconditionally dislike milk, however. Milk has a near perfect balance of macronutrients—protein, fat, and carbohydrates—beneficial conjugated fatty acids, calcium, and vitamin D, despite some people's intolerance to it. If you know you have an issue with lactose, the sugar in milk or casein, the protein in milk, and you feel better without it, then leave out. Keep in mind that most hard cheeses are lactose-free and are low in carbohydrates. Milk, by virtue of being from an animal, will have some hormones, but organic milk decreases the hormone load. If dairy works for you, keep it, but buy organic.

Nonfat, 2 percent, or whole milk plain, kefirs (fermented milk); unsweetened regular and Greek yogurts; and hard cheeses can still fit into a lower-carbohydrate diet but are tougher to fit into a VLC diet of fewer than 50 grams per day.

*Goal: Unsweetened milk, yogurt and kefir—zero to two servings per day; hard cheeses—one to three ounces per day.*

**6. Reduce high FODMAPs, nuts, seeds, and legumes.** Legumes provide protein, fiber, and carbohydrates; some contain small amounts of fats. Humans don't have the enzyme to break apart galactans, the sugars in legumes, so even a healthy gut may get gassy. My preference is to remove legumes first before nuts and seeds. Sprouted legumes may be easier to digest.

Nuts and seeds provide healthy fats, some protein, and a small amount of carbohydrates, in addition to other minerals—a nice balance. They do not drastically elevate blood sugars, and they help to quell your hunger pangs. Some nuts are harder for some bellies, so eat ten or fewer nuts at a time, unless your belly agrees with more. Of course, if you know you have a nut allergy, including any kind of swelling, rash, or difficulty breathing, then avoid those nuts.

*Goal: Omit legumes first, then limit nuts and seeds. If GI is not an issue, nuts and seeds can stay in a low-carb diet.*

**7. Reduce other fruits and vegetables.** Decrease only the high-FODMAP fruits and vegetables if they bother your belly. I prefer to reduce these last, since many are high in many nutrients. Keep the low FODMAP fruits and vegetables since they are also high in nutrients and low in fermentable sugars. If you know for sure that a high-FODMAP fruit or vegetable bothers you, such as apples or onions, go ahead and limit it sooner.

Remember, the FODMAPs approach is to lower the total amount of FODMAPs; reducing other less-nutrient-dense carbohydrates first may allow you to eat more higher-FODMAP nutrient-dense fruits and veggies. The goal of lowering by layers is to reduce carbohydrates by nutrient density, monitoring your symptoms along the way and not reducing more than you need. If your belly and bathroom visits are okay and your blood sugar and weight are moving in the right direction, let that be your guide. The first layers are the least nutritious foods, moving down to the last layer of FODMAPs: fruits and vegetables.

Keep in mind, healing a sensitive gut includes not just removing the antagonizing foods but making other lifestyle changes and possibly taking supplements to boost nutrient deficiencies and reduce inflammation. Some supplements, though, have antimicrobial effects. Consider a consultation with a qualified nutritionist, who can help you consider all options to help heal.

---

**Summary of Lowering Carbohydrates by Layers**

1. Reduce sweets, desserts, and concentrated sources of sugar.
2. Reduce gluten-containing foods.
3. Reduce all other grains, except sprouted or sourdough breads, if you choose to keep them.
4. Reduce tuberous root vegetables and all other starchy vegetables.
5. Reduce dairy unless you limited it earlier.
6. Reduce high-FODMAP legumes, then nuts, and seeds, unless you've identified a culprit sooner.
7. Reduce high-FODMAP fruits and vegetables, unless you've identified a culprit sooner.

---

## How Did You Do?

Okay, time to pull out those two days of carb counting I asked you to do a few sections back. How does your usual day fit in? Think about your cardiac and GI-related risk factors and which approach might fit you best. If your usual intake is 250 grams a day with few sources of fiber, even just cutting your total intake by 50 grams can have positive effects, especially if you look closer at the type of carbohydrates.

These two approaches of reducing carbohydrates—counting grams or removing in layers—are not set in stone. I have many clients who have gray areas regarding how much and which carbohydrates they keep. If you can't imagine life without some sweets and can handle one cookie a day, then go for it. If you're counting carbs, count it in your allowance or just substitute it for a grain. If you've struggled for years with weight loss, try eating fewer than 50 grams a day to jump start your progress. Then gradually increase your carbohydrate gram allowance by 10 to 25 grams a day, with primarily nutrient-dense choices, until you find a spot where you can comfortably lose or maintain your weight.

Trying one of these approaches, however, gives you some system to your day and helps you stick with it. Consider seeing a nutritionist or registered dietitian who can help fine-tune your changes, check that you're eating the right amount of protein and fat, help with behavior changes, and also take a look at your medications and supplements.

Most importantly, understand the connection between your carbohydrate intake, your blood sugar, the insulin you produce, and your GI health. As your awareness and knowledge increase, shuffling your carbs around to suit your needs will become second nature.

## Key Takeaways

1. Removing carbohydrates in layers, starting with the least-nutrient-dense foods and moving up to the most-nutrient-dense carbs is one approach to lowering your carb intake, helping to improve blood sugars and also helping GI distress.
2. If you know of a food that you are intolerant or allergic to, avoid it sooner.
3. This approach has as much wiggle room as you want to give it. You can be strict or lenient depending on your symptoms; it is largely driven by nutrient density.
4. If you do not choose to fully omit the grains, try to limit to a maximum of two servings per day.

# Part 6

## Loose Ends

# 27

# Some Final Thoughts

## *What Do Our Organs Use for Fuel?*

Are carbohydrates really the preferred fuel for our body, or is it one that modern society has become used to and addicted to because of its overabundance? This question really reaches the heart of the matter, understanding the preferred fuel for our body and its parts. Humans as a species have some general preferences for fuel sources, but again, one size does not fit all, nor every circumstance.

Our organs and cells use different fuel sources for different situations, with some even being quite specific to an individual amino acid. For example, the small intestine cells known as *enterocytes* use the amino acid glutamine proportionally more than other cells in the body. Epigenetics may influence your preferred fuel for your body and how that plays out into the best balanced diet for you.

## What Fuel Does It Take to Go from Here to There?

Here are some basics about energy utilization. Unlike fat, glucose is anaerobic; it doesn't need oxygen to be present for our skeletal muscle cells to use it for energy. If it did, as mentioned earlier, the world record for the hundred-meter dash would not be less than ten seconds. So, yes, glucose does the job faster, delivering ATP to skeletal muscles with less oxygen for quick bursts of energy and at exercise intensities above 85 percent of our muscle's maximum effort.

However, for the long haul, and for daily living when there is more oxygen available, fat is the preferred fuel source for skeletal muscle. In fact, as you are reading this, you're burning a mixture of fuels: glucose and fat. This is not new; it's the way the body has always worked. Most organs can use glucose, fat or fatty acids, or ketones for fuel. (We'll talk about ketones next.)

Cardiologists recognize that because the heart uses so much oxygen, it likes fatty acids best for fuel, up to 65 percent of its calories, especially when you are not exercising. The heart is adaptable and changes its fuel source according to its needs; in the case of a heart attack, for example, when less oxygen is present, the heart will use glucose. The heart actually stores small amounts of glycogen as glucose. A healthy, fit heart, however, will actually use lactate from the lactic acid released by muscles to fuel itself, even as much as glucose. (It's not the lactate part of lactic acid that is the cause of pain and fatigue, but the hydrogen or acid part.) But don't forget: too many carbohydrates in the diet may actually cause a broken heart, or at least an inflamed one.

## Do Some Organs Prefer Glucose?

The brain, red blood cells, and the kidney use glucose first. Perhaps we notice this best by our mood swings when our blood sugars go up and down. Our brain doesn't have a reserve supply of glycogen or glucose storage, like the liver or even as our heart does. The brain relies upon a direct, almost second-to-second flow from our bloodstream.

Although the brain probably uses glucose best, it can also use ketones quite well. Ketones are a by-product of fat metabolism. Even though the brain is made primarily of fat and water, it cannot use fatty acids directly for fuel. However, just because the brain uses glucose efficiently doesn't mean that more is better; nor do we need to eat 3,000 calories of it each day. In fact, research is showing that excessive sugar and carbohydrates contribute to *glycation*, an inflammatory process of proteins building up in the brain that is related to cognitive changes, including Alzheimer's disease. Remember, a good marker for potential glycation is the hemoglobin A1C blood test.

With exercise intensities greater than 85 percent of maximum oxygen consumption, muscle cells must use glycogen stores because glycogen is more efficient. Fitter athletes demonstrate efficient fuel usage best. When they increase fats in their diets and decrease carbohydrates, they can slow glycogen loss by increasing how efficiently their muscles burn certain triglycerides stored in them. Decreasing carbohydrates may help our bodies use our fatty acids more efficiently for fuel while also better managing our glucose and glycogen stores.

## Key Takeaways

1. Fatty acids are the preferred fuel source for muscles, including the heart. Fatty acids require the presence of oxygen to be used for fuel.
2. The brain prefers glucose for fuel but can also easily use ketones. Glucose can be converted to energy quicker with less oxygen—faster than fatty acids.
3. One of the benefits of reducing carbohydrates and increasing dietary fat is allowing the body to use fatty acids as a fuel source first more readily. Trained endurance athletes do this best.

# 28

# Ketosis: Friend or Foe?

We produce ketones as a by-product of fat metabolism for fuel when carbohydrates are not available. Ketones have gotten a bad rap because typically people think of diabetic ketosis, which can be a life-threatening emergency.

Diabetic ketoacidosis—where the pancreas makes too little insulin—occurs in type 1 diabetes or late-stage type 2 diabetes. With deficient insulin, the most predominant ketone, beta-hydroxybutyrate (B-OHB) rises in the blood to 15 to 25 mM, a very acidic state and not one the kidneys and body can maintain for long. No doubt, it's dangerous.

We safely produce ketones, however, during low carbohydrate intake and starvation as a different fuel alternative. Ketone production is just a different metabolic fuel pathway and one that our ancestors likely existed on for millennia. Ketosis from reduction of carbohydrates in an otherwise healthy body produces much lower levels of ketones than diabetic ketosis and is not dangerous. The primary blood ketone we produce in nondiabetic ketosis is also beta-hydroxybutyrate. B-OHB blood levels can rise above 0.5 milli molar (mM), which is much lower than in diabetic ketoacidosis. Eating even just 20 grams a day of carbohydrates only rarely stimulates ketones above 3 mM. Taking carbohydrate reduction a bit further to total starvation, blood B-OHB may increase to 5 mM, which is still far lower than in diabetic acidosis.

In nondiabetic ketosis the brain shifts gears and gets more of its energy from ketones, decreasing the need for glucose and insulin, especially with carbohydrate levels less than 50 grams per day. In fact, research shows that B-OHB may be more efficient for producing ATP than glucose. Also, keep in mind that B-OHB does stimulate a little insulin, but marginally—much less than protein and far less than carbohydrates. Fat stimulates no insulin. For all the heat that fat gets, it can't be blamed for too much insulin.

Ketosis essentially gives humans the flexibility to deal with famine or major shifts in available food, except that the plan probably wasn't for us to be challenged with exorbitant amounts of carbohydrates every day, more than four times what people first consumed. Potentially, our daily carbohydrate intake today exhausts the beta cells of the pancreas and in the end makes the body not so adaptable.

Keep in mind that the ketogenic diet was the primary treatment for certain kinds of epilepsy in children, before Big Pharma came along. Some treatment programs still use it. Many people who eat a VLC diet and go into ketosis are able to reduce and stop diabetes and cholesterol medications. This approach strays from the traditional wisdom, and it's hard for some health professionals to accept that such profound changes could occur without drugs for such metabolically resistant people.

Although hunter-gatherers existed in ketosis for varying periods of times without negative consequences, the question still remains: Does long-term ketosis in today's world pose health risks—not from the metabolic state itself, which research shows is safe, considering our ancestors, but more from the potential risk of fewer fermentable carbohydrates to help build a strong, immune protective gut. Our world now carries a greater toxic load, and we may need greater gut protection than our ancestors did.

For more information on understanding low-carbohydrate eating in other cultures, and ketosis associated with low-carbohydrate diets, see the works of Jeff Volk, RD, PhD, and Stephen Phinney, MD, PhD—two researchers on the forefront of this field who have followed low-carbohydrate eating for over twenty-five years apiece.

## Key Takeaways

1. Nondiabetic ketosis is not dangerous and is a metabolic state that many hunter gatherer cultures existed on, depending on the season.
2. Ketosis is a shift in fuel usage because of fewer available carbohy-

drates. The body produces ketones from fatty acids. Ketones are a safe and efficient fuel source for the brain and muscles.

3. Diabetic ketosis is a dangerous place to be. It produces much higher levels of ketones than nondiabetic ketosis, primarily because of inadequate insulin to transport glucose to the cell.

4. Ketosis is not a new phenomenon; it has been used to treat various conditions, including epilepsy, for decades and now quite clearly can quickly promote weight loss, and improve blood sugars and blood lipids that contribute to metabolic syndrome. In certain individuals who have more weight to lose or who are metabolically resistant, ketosis may be the best option.

5. The risks of long-term ketosis in today's society if it sacrifices gut-beneficial carbs is unknown. Each person's health risks must be considered.

# 29

# One Last Thought: What's Evolution Got to Do with It?

Has the human genetic code changed much in millions of years? Probably not, but maybe a little, which is important to keep in mind when understanding varying levels of carbohydrates in certain lifestyles many years ago. The Inuit people in the Canadian Arctic ate very few carbohydrates while the Kitava people in New Guinea still enjoy up to 60 percent of their calories from carbohydrates.

Harvard-trained anthropologist Vilhjalmur Stefansson lived with and studied the Inuit people in the early 1900s and then shared with Bellevue Hospital his positive experience of living a year eating low carb—fewer than 50 grams a day. In contrast, the Kitava people from New Guinea continue to eat a high-carbohydrate diet, just as their ancestors did. They have been studied because of their low cardiac risk markers. Their diet includes root vegetables (sweet potatoes), fruit, vegetables, fish, and coconut. Note, however, that they receive protein from the fish and fat from the coconut.

Despite history showing early man living very well on few carbohydrates, humans are blessed with the ability to break down amylose, one of the starch molecules we met earlier. Anthropology studies show that people in cultures that eat the most starch have more AMY1, the amylase enzyme secreted in our saliva that gets first stab at breaking down starch. We also make amylase in the pancreas, Amy2, but less variation in number occurs with Amy2. Having more than two copies of a gene is called *copy number variation (CNV)*. Geneticists believe that eating more starch didn't trigger more amylase genes to appear in early man, but rather those who had the extra amylase survived better and produced more kids—an example of natural selection or survival of the fittest. A higher number of AMY1 genes helps digestion of starchy foods and may protect against some intestinal disease. Knowing how many of these genes you have requires genetic testing, perhaps not necessary but interesting to know and helping further explain some of our epigenetic influences.

Even though gene number variation is thought to exist to help with fertility, to keep the generations going and not necessarily longevity, scientists believed it was uncommon, but as the human genome was studied more, it appeared more. I suspect there is a lot more we don't know about our genes that is associated with which foods work best with our body. A great example of medicine moving toward using epigenetics and nutragenomics is demonstrated by the results of research done by King's College in London looking at the number of amylase genes and the incidence of obesity. Several different studies including 149 Swedish families, 481 Swedish families and 927 twins from the Twins UK—the United Kingdom's largest twin registry—show similar patterns in obesity related to the amylase gene. A significant increase in risk of obesity was seen with the most versus the least number of amylase genes. Similar results have been found in other countries. The mechanism is unclear but may be related to undigested starch in those people with fewer amylase genes entering the gut, changing the gut environment and leading to insulin resistance, increasing the risk for obesity.

## Carb Food for Thought!

My guess is that most people don't stay up at night contemplating their starch genes or what we are or are not designed to eat. I must be in the right profession, because I do wonder about such things. I wonder why we lack the enzymes to digest some of the more prevalent sugars found in carbohydrates in today's food supply, such as fructans and galactans. My best guess is maybe we're not supposed to eat a lot of them. Some of their fermentable sugars may be beneficial, but again each of us is different.

Medicine doesn't know the perfect diet for each of us, but we know characteristics of foods that are beneficial and characteristics that are not. We also know that components of food may affect our genes, our cells, and ultimately our immune system and health. The cultures that thrived on both low- and high-carb diets had something in common: no triple mocha lattes, no soda, no McDonald's or Dunkin' Donuts, no high fructose corn syrup—no daily intake of acellular, refined, manipulated, processed carbs!

Yes, there may be variations in the amounts of carbohydrates in different cultures, with some doing quite well for generations, probably in ketosis, and other cultures eating higher amounts of carbohydrates, but they are from root vegetables, nonstarchy vegetables, or fruits—all nutrient-dense! And most likely they did not eat over 500 grams of them a day or take acid blockers or other medications that change the gut environment. Also, hunter-gatherers were the ultimate endurance athletes. They needed to have a fuel source for the long run because the amounts of carbohydrates we have today just weren't available. Eating fewer carbs and higher amounts of fats enabled them to utilize their fat stores efficiently, saving their glycogen until they really needed it.

Geneticists speculate that the reason we develop certain gene changes is to better the chances of making new humans. For that to happen, our body understands that the evolutionary change must include a shift toward, for example, additional nutrients, not just a convenient gene or enzyme to prevent harm from our poor choices. Although medicine and science today seem to be focused on longevity, our environment and lifestyles present us with far more toxins and contaminants than previous generations. That convenient gene to prevent harm from poor choices would be mighty handy. Some people seem to be more protected than others.

So, what's my final word on carbohydrates? Carbs by any name are seductive. We eat far more than we intend or realize. They have taken over our daily meal choices and food supply. For many, our organs can't keep up. Research and history suggest that we are supposed to have some carbohydrates in our diet, but the amount is probably different for each of us. My educated guess goes back to my million-dollar question about finding a balance of carbohydrates that is low enough to keep blood sugar and insulin levels healthy, while also high enough and with the right type to maintain a healthy gut and thereby a healthy immune system.

Ultimately, you know your body better than anyone, so tune

in and listen. To live a healthy, functional life in the twenty-first century, we need all the protection we can get. Processed foods, especially processed carbohydrates, may have inflammatory effects because of their impact on insulin and our gut flora. They seduce us and disguise themselves as healthy because we are infatuated with their taste, texture, and feel. But don't be fooled. Your body knows better and will eventually tell you. Pay attention to your red flags. Carbobesity and carbo-gut can be avoided and managed by finding your sweet spot of carbohydrate tolerance—the amount and type that fit you best.

## Key Takeaways

1. Humans have the starch gene enzyme amylase to break down the starch amylose. Some people have more than others. But given the presence of the gene in our species, we're probably supposed to have some amylose.
2. Studies on nutrigenomics are revealing that people with fewer amylose genes have a greater risk for obesity.
3. One thing all early cultures had in common regardless of their carbohydrate content was the absence of refined, manufactured carbs. Manufactured carbohydrates are low in nutrients, raise blood sugars, and may promote gut dysbiosis.
4. Given the greater toxic load that our world carries today, finding that optimal level of carbohydrates is probably the result of maintaining a balance of healthy blood sugar, insulin, and a healthy, well-protected gut.

# Appendix 1

## Sample Days

## Sample Day of 50 Grams of Carbohydrates or Less

*Aim for 10 to 15 grams of carbs per meal from nonstarchy vegetables and lower-carbohydrate fruits, such as berries.*

### Breakfast: 5–10 grams
2 eggs
2 slices Canadian bacon
½ cup sautéed mushrooms and 1 cup spinach; use organic, salted broth to sauté.

### Lunch: 10 grams
1 cup broth—chicken, beef, or fish
5 oz. chicken, pork, or meat
1 cup cruciferous vegetables (broccoli, cauliflower)
1 cup greens with olive oil and vinegar

### Dinner: 16 grams
5 oz. roast chicken
1 cup kale sautéed with olive oil and garlic
½ cup berries with 2–3 Tbsp. unsweetened whipped cream

### Snacks: Choose two
10 almonds (2.5 grams)
4 black or green olives (2–3 grams)

¼ cup avocado slices (3 grams)
1 oz. hard cheddar cheese (0 grams)

## Sample Day of 50 to 100 Grams

*Count and add the following foods to the 50-gram-carb day to keep in the desired carbohydrate range.*

Two ½ cups nonstarchy vegetable (10 grams)
One starchy vegetable (10–15 grams)
½–¾ cup berries (15 grams)
½ oz. 70 percent dark chocolate (8 grams)

## Sample Day of 75 to 150 Grams

*Continue to add the following choices. Aim for a minimum of five servings of nonstarchy vegetables. Refer to the "How Much Lives Where" chapter for a reminder of a serving size, or read the label.*

1 cup nonstarchy vegetable (5 grams)
⅛ cup nuts of choice (5 grams)
1 fruit (15 grams)
1 starchy vegetable (15 grams)
1 grain (15 grams)
6-8 oz dairy—unsweetened yogurt or milk (12 grams)

\* \* \*

If you choose to eat beyond 150 grams of carbohydrates a day, keep track of your blood sugars, weight, and belly patterns, and continue to add the above foods. You will have room for limited grains and two to three dairy choices, as tolerated. See Appendix 2 for a summary of goals.

# Appendix 2

# The Short and Long of It: Carb Goals

For improved blood sugars, weight control, and belly symptoms, consider the following summary recommendations with short- and long-term goals of foods based on their nutritional value and their effects on blood sugar. Use the seven layers for removing carbohydrates if you have GI issues, but also consider these goals. You be the judge of your GI symptoms if you know of a culprit food that needs to be removed sooner.

For plant choices, whether fruit or vegetables, aim to include red, orange, yellow, green, and blue-purple.

*Short term* indicates at least two weeks to either help jump start a weight-loss effort or determine a food's effect on your gut. Restricting certain foods may be necessary for up to six to eight weeks before gut improvements are seen; best results are usually achieved when working with a qualified nutritionist. If you are restricting carbohydrates so that you are in ketosis, check with a qualified nutritionist and your physician to help determine that you're meeting your nutritional needs, as well as long-term plans.

For the *long term*, after initially removing certain carbohydrates or reducing to a very low carbohydrates (VLC) diet, you may want to increase your carbohydrates back to a level that helps you maintain your positive changes. You do not need to be perfect with these long-term goals, but they are goals to practice *most of the time*. You can decide on a time frequency that allows you to have more freedom but it should be practiced with the intention that these long term changes are for a lifetime. Most importantly, keep track of the important risk markers that are influenced by your carbohydrate intake, including blood sugars, triglycerides, waist circumference, and GI comfort.

131

In the following lists, which instruct you on how much to eat to meet short- and long-term goals, an asterisk (*) indicates a high-FODMAP food. See the Monash University link for more on FODMAPs: http://www.med.monash.edu/cecs/gastro/fodmap/.

# Sugar

**Short-term.** Minimal, if any. Eat foods without sugars on the label or at least farther down on the ingredient listing.

**Long-term.** Minimal. Only if you can maintain a healthy blood sugar, weight, and GI are small amounts then allowed. Set limits; pay attention to FODMAPs as needed.

*Agave, beet sugar, brown sugar, syrup cane-juice crystals, caramel, carob syrup, corn syrup, dextran, dextrose, fructose, fructans, glucose, *honey, *high fructose corn syrup, inverted sugar, *lactose, maltose, *maltitol, maltodextrin, *mannitol, *sorbitol, turbino sugar, maple syrup, *molasses, *xylitol.

Soda, juices, candy, pastries, cookies, cakes, pies, etc.

# Whole Grains

*1 serving, 75–110 calories, 15 grams carbs*

**Short-term.** Consider removal; first gluten-containing, then gluten-free. No room for them in a VLC diet.

**Long-term.** Limit to zero to two servings per day, depending on blood sugars and GI symptoms. You may be able to handle more, but let these markers be your guide.

**Gluten-free grains:** Amaranth, arrowroot, bean flours *(garbanzo, fava, Romano), buckwheat, corn, fava beans, flax seed, garbanzo beans (chickpeas), hominy, mesquite flour, millet, montina flour, nut flour and nut meals, oats, pea flour, potato flour or potato starch, quinoa, rice (all forms), rice bran, sago, sorghum flour, *soybeans and soy flour, tapioca (manioc, cassava, yucca), teff flour.

**Gluten-containing grains:** *Barley, bulgur, chapatti flour (atta), couscous, dinkel or spelt, durum, einkorn, emmer, farina, farro, fu gluten flour, graham flour, kamut, *malt, matzoh meal, oats, orzo, *rye, seitan, semolina, textured vegetable protein, triticale, *wheat (bran, germ, starch), any gluten containing sourdough flour.

## Starchy Vegetables

*1 serving, 80 calories, 15 grams carbs*
**Short-term.** Consider omitting; no room for them in a VLC diet.
**Long-term.** Zero to two servings per day.
1 cup acorn squash, cubed; 1 cup beets, cubed; 1 cup butternut squash, cubed; 1 cup celery root, cubed; ⅓ cup Plantain (½ whole); ½ medium potato (purple, red, yellow); ½ cup potatoes, mashed; ½ cup root vegetables (parsnip, rutabaga); ½ medium sweet potato.

## Legumes

*1 serving, 110 calories, 15 grams carbs, 7 grams protein*
**Short-term.** Zero to one serving per day; no room for them in a VLC diet.
**Long-term.** Zero to two servings per day.
*¾ cup bean soups; *½ cup black soybeans (cooked); *½ cup dried beans (kidney, baked, lentils, peas [cooked]); *½ cup edamame (cooked); *⅓ cup hummus or other bean dips; ½ cup green peas (cooked).

## Nuts and Seeds

*1 serving, 45 calories, 4 grams fat, 2–6 grams carbs*
**Short-term.** One to four servings per day.
**Long-term.** Two to four servings per day.
6 almonds; 2 Brazil nuts; *6 cashews; 1 Tbsp. chia seeds; 3 Tbsp. coconut, dried flakes (unsweetened); 2 Tbsp. flaxseed, ground; 5 hazelnuts; 1 Tbsp. hemp seeds; 6 mixed nuts; ½ Tbsp. nut and seed butters; 10 peanuts; 4 pecan halves; 1 Tbsp. pine nuts; *16 pistachios; 1 Tbsp. pumpkin seeds; 2 Tbsp. soy nuts; 1 Tbsp. sesame seeds; 1 Tbsp. sunflower seed kernels; 4 walnut halves.

## Dairy/Alternatives

*1 serving, 50–100 calories, 12 grams carbs, 7 grams protein*
**Short-term.** Omit except for hard cheeses and sour cream.
**Long-term.** One to three servings per day.

*8 oz. buttermilk; 8 oz. kefir, plain (unsweetened); *8 oz. milk (cow, goat, sheep); 8 oz. lactose-free milk, yogurt; 4 oz. milk (hemp, oat [unsweetened]); *8 oz. milk alternatives (coconut, nut soy [unsweetened]); *6 oz. yogurt, plain (unsweetened);
*4 oz. yogurt (Greek), plain (unsweetened); ¼ cup cottage cheese; 3 Tbsp. sour cream (less than 2 grams carbs); 1 oz. cheeses (Brie, Camembert, cheddar, feta, mozzarella, Parmesan (less than 1 gram carbs).

## Fruits

*No sugars added; avoid juices and limit dried fruit: 1 serving, 60 calories, 15 grams carbs*
**Short-term.** Zero to two servings per day.
**Long-term.** Two to three servings per day.
*Small apple; ½ cup unsweetened applesauce; *apricots, fresh; ½ banana;
¾ cup *blackberries or blueberries; *boysenberry (29 grams carbs in ½ cup); *12 cherries; *½ grapefruit; 15 grapes; 1 kiwi; ½ small mango; 1 cup melon (all [*watermelon]); *1 small nectarine; 1 small orange; 1 cup papaya; *1 small peach, 1 small pear; *½ persimmon; ¾ cup pineapple; 2 small plums; 1 small pomegranate;
1 cup raspberries; 1¼ cup strawberries; 2 small tangerines.

## Nonstarchy Vegetables

*½ cup cooked, 1 cup raw, 25 calories, 5 grams carbs*
**Short-term.** Five to ten servings per day.
**Long-term.** Five to ten servings per day.
*Artichoke, arugula, *asparagus, bamboo shoots, bok choy, broccoflower, broccoli, brussels sprouts, cabbage, carrots, *cauliflower, celery, chard/Swiss chard, chives, endive, escarole, eggplant, fennel, *garlic, green beans, greens (beet, collard, dandelion, kale, mustard, turnip), horseradish, jicama, kohlrabi, *leeks, lettuce (all), *mushrooms, okra, *onions, parsley, peppers (all), *pumpkin, radicchio, radishes, salsa, scallions, sea vegetables, *shallots, *snap peas/snow peas, spinach, sprouts (all), squash (delicata, pumpkin, spaghetti, yellow, zucchini), tomato, tomato juice, turnips, vegetable juice, water chestnuts, watercress.

## Fats and Oils

*Minimally refined, cold-pressed, organic, non-GMO preferred, 1 serving, 45 calories, 5 grams fat, 0 carbs*
**Short-term.** Four to nine servings per day.
**Long-term.** Four to nine servings per day; may be higher depending on energy needs.

2 Tbsp. avocado; 1 tsp. butter (2 tsp. whipped); 1 square chocolate, dark (70  percent or higher coca; 1 square = 7 grams); 1½ Tbsp. *coconut milk, regular (canned); 1 tsp. oils, cooking (butter, coconut [virgin], grapeseed, olive [extra virgin]); 1 tsp. oils, salad (almond, canola, flaxseed, grapeseed, olive [extra virgin], rice bran, high oleic safflower or sunflower, sesame, walnut).

## Protein

1-oz. serving, 35–75 calories, 7 grams protein, 0 carbohydrates; preferably, grass-fed, organic, non-GMO.
**Short- and long-term.** 1–1.5 grams/kg optimal weight for most people, or about 50 to 130 grams a day (may vary with high levels of activity). Aim for 20 to 30 grams per meal, 5 to 10 grams per snack (1 oz. equals 7 grams of protein).

1 oz. cheese; *¼ cup cottage cheese; 1 egg or 2 egg whites; ⅔ cup egg substitute; 1 oz. feta cheese; 2 Tbsp. Parmesan cheese

1 oz. fish/shellfish: halibut, herring, mackerel, salmon (wild), sardines, tuna, etc.

1 oz. meat: beef, buffalo, elk, lamb, venison, other wild game

1 oz. poultry: chicken, Cornish hen, turkey.

## Plant Protein

*1-oz. serving, 45 calories, 7 grams protein. If you are a strict vegan, it's harder to lower carbohydrates but possible. However, since all food sources are coming from foods with more carbohydrates, it's more challenging to address GI sensitivities.*

*1 oz. burger alternatives: mushroom, soy, veggie (10 grams carbs); *3 Tbsp. Miso (14 grams carbs); *¼ cup natto (6 grams carbs); *½ cup tofu (2.3 carbs); ½ cup tempeh (8 grams carbs).

# Appendix 3

## Okay, What Can I Eat?
## Ten Keepers and More

Just the thought of eating fewer carbohydrates may make some people anxious and depressed; after all, these are many of our favorite foods that I'm asking you to reduce. My experience is that most people see such profound positive changes—whether in the form of weight control, improvements in cardiac markers, or improvements in GI symptoms—that any reduction in carbohydrates is welcomed and well worth the tradeoff. However, I'm not suggesting it is easy. It takes focus, determination, and motivation. But more often than not, my clients much prefer the benefits their body receives from these changes versus the short-term gratification that excessive carbohydrates may provide. Also, once you learn how to handle your trigger situations, such as stress, and incorporate exercise, you will see that a setback need not steer you into black-and-white mode and forget all that you've learned.

Also, because the foods you are allowed to eat are more filling after you get into the swing of it, your more natural hunger patterns will emerge. Without insulin controlling your dramatic shifts in blood sugar, a lower-carbohydrate diet typically better regulates your appetite. It's not as hard as you might think. Your choices become almost second nature. Most people have improved energy, sleep, and confidence. Ultimately, don't you want to feel better?

With seemingly so many foods being high in carbohydrates, what's left to eat? Here's a list of foods that you are able to eat in satisfying, though not limitless, portions in a diet of 75 grams per day of carbohydrates or higher. Enjoy!

**All nonstarchy vegetables.** Stroll the produce aisles and get to know all the different vegetables that are out there; it is an education in realizing vegetables are a big world with many options. It's not just carrots and peas. Choose from the rainbow-red, orange, yellow, green, and blue-purple varieties. Often people find that once they reduce sweets, their palate begins to become more accepting of a variety of flavors that vegetables offer. *Aim for half of your plate to be filled with nonstarchy veggies.*

**All fruits, especially berries.** Blueberries, black raspberries, raspberries, and strawberries all offer many nutrients and phytochemicals and taste good. Top a warm bowl of berries with 1–2 Tbsp. of real whipped cream and it's hard to feel deprived. Blueberries always top any list of foods with high levels of protective phytochemicals, and they are low in FODMAPs, so they are easy on the belly.

**Eggs.** Practically zero carbohydrates and nearly the perfect protein, eggs offer a host of nutrients, including vitamins A, D, and E; riboflavin; folic acid; and choline, which is important for the brain. Yes, eggs have cholesterol, but remember that we need cholesterol for all of our cells, and our body regulates its production with what we eat. Research strongly questions the "lipid hypothesis" as the primary factor in heart disease; rather it points to inflammation from a variety of factors in our lives as being the primary cause. If you are eating fewer carbohydrates from healthy choices and your risk markers are moving in the right direction, and you're not allergic to eggs, enjoy. Eggs mix well with a variety of foods, including vegetables, and cook in five minutes.

**Avocados.** Avocados are the new healthy, once forbidden food. Actually, avocados have always been healthy, but they are certainly reinventing themselves. Avocados have healthy fats, are lower in carbohydrates, and are satisfying. Slice half an avocado on a salad or even eat it plain. Mash them with cherry tomatoes or your favorite salsa. Once you've cut into an avocado, save the remaining portion in a small covered container and add a small amount of lemon or lime juice to help prevent browning.

**Meat, poultry, and fish.** All animal and fish proteins provide us with all essential amino acids, so they're a protein bargain. We don't need the whole animal but a few ounces throughout the day. Best to divide protein evenly between meals and snacks. We don't use the protein from eating a 12-ounce steak all at once nearly as well as when we eat 2 to 4 ounces at a time.

**Unsweetened yogurts and kefirs.** It's the added sugars in yogurts and kefirs that can get you into trouble. Plain, unsweetened Greek and regular yogurts offer calcium and protein, and conjugated fats if you eat the two percent or whole versions, as well as healthy bacteria for your belly, depending on the brand. Add your own fruit, vanilla, or cinnamon. If you eat dairy daily, choose organic. Of note: the whey protein in milk is thought to be of the best quality protein; because of the availability of the branched chain amino acids, particularly leucine.

**Hard cheese.** Hard cheeses are low in lactose and high in protein, calcium, and conjugated fats. If you are not intolerant, they are a convenient snack or add-on to a meal. Again, it's the carbohydrates, usually refined, that we eat with cheeses that are damaging. Depending on your tolerance, enjoy 1–2 ounces a day.

**Nuts and seeds.** All nuts are generally lower in carbohydrates and contain healthy fats and small amounts of protein, making nuts a satisfying snack or add-on to a meal. Cashews and pistachios are higher in FODMAPs, so be careful if you are sensitive. Enjoy nuts and seeds every day and enjoy all varieties: almonds, cashews, peanuts, walnuts, pistachios, and Brazil nuts. Seeds include chia, hemp, pumpkin, sesame, and sunflower.

**Nut and seed butters.** Like their whole counterparts, nut butters—such as almond or peanut—or SunButter can be a tasty treat on vegetables or a slice of sprouted bread or just by the spoonful.

**Dark chocolate greater than 70 percent cacao.** Some bellies do better than others with chocolate, so be careful with quantity. Dark chocolate really does have medicinal properties, including improvements in blood pressure and blood sugar; research suggests the benefits are related to the flavonoids. Try different manufacturers; not all 70 percent chocolate tastes alike. Because dark chocolate is lower in sugar and actually provides some fiber, it can help nip a sugar craving in the bud quite nicely. For maximum savoriness and enjoyment, allow it to melt in your mouth—no biting.

**Healthy fats.** Flavor your foods with small to moderate amounts of healthy fats, including olive oil, coconut oil, whole milk dairy, ghee, and even butter. Vegetable oils, especially heavily processed oils, oxidize at higher heats and may be detrimental to our bodies. Better to fry with ghee, coconut oil, or butter; sautéing in olive oil is okay, too.

**Whipped cream and sour cream.** We're not talking a bowl of these creams, but yes, you can have a few tablespoons on berries or vegetables, or however you like. Research doesn't show that saturated fat is harmful or raises cardiac risk or mortality. It's more the carbohydrates usually eaten with those saturated fats that are damaging, possibly because of the influence of insulin. And if your risk markers and symptoms are moving in the right direction, then enjoy these in limited amounts.

**Oatmeal, quinoa, and tuberous vegetables.** Although these foods are high in carbohydrates, if your carbohydrate allowance allows for them given your risk markers and goals, then oatmeal, quinoa, sweet potatoes, and sprouted breads are your healthiest options for both blood sugar and belly concerns. Oatmeal can be filling, can be purchased gluten free, is lower in FODMAPs, and may be beneficial to blood sugar. Quinoa is gluten free, low in FODMAPs, and offers a high protein for a grain; people also tend to eat quinoa in smaller quantities than rice or pastas. Tuberous vegetables are naturally portion-controlled when cooked and purchased as singles; aim for a small sweet potato. Sprouted breads may be lower in gluten and fructans. Celiac patients should still avoid sprouted breads unless they are labeled gluten-free, but some nonceliac gluten-sensitive people can still eat sprouted wheat.

**Spices.** Use spices to spice up your palate. Spices by their nature often have a concentrated flavor that is not sweet. They have unique flavors that challenge other taste buds and can help curb a sweet tooth. Because they are from plants, they contain a variety of different phytochemicals that are beneficial to our bodies. Consider using cinnamon, nutmeg, vanilla, unsweetened cocoa powder, peppers, turmeric, or curry powder on foods of your choice. Experiment: a dash of cinnamon can liven up a meal.

## Easy, Smart Snacks

Snacks are foods we eat between meals and can greatly help control mealtime portion sizes by preventing our blood sugar from dropping too low. But remember, part of why our blood sugar drops is from excessive refined carbohydrates and poor insulin regulation.

Just as with meals, aim for snacks to be well balanced in nutrients with a lower glycemic index/load. Calories do count, but focus more on the balance and the carb content. One hundred to 300 calories and a carbohydrate content of 0 to 15 grams is just the right amount for most people to notice an improvement in blood sugar but also provides satiety and contentment before the next meal. Also remember that MMC in our belly needs a break between meals and snacks to help keep proper motility, so no grazing.

- 1 Tbsp. or other nut butter alone or with apple slices (one small apple).
- 10–20 of any nuts: mixed, almonds, walnuts, cashews, pistachios.
- ½ cup Greek or regular, plain, 0 percent, 2 percent, or whole yogurt with your choice of a handful of berries, 10 nuts, 2 tsp. of seeds, or a sprinkle of cinnamon or vanilla.
- 1- to 2-oz. roll-up of any meat or poultry, with several large leafy greens (spinach, kale, romaine) and 1–2 tsp. unsweetened mustard of your choice.
- 1 oz. of any hard cheese without crackers, or rolled up with greens of your choice.
- 1 slice sprouted bread with ½ sliced avocado.
- ½ cup of raw, sliced vegetables with ½ avocado mashed with your favorite salsa or cherry tomatoes and 1 tsp. lime juice.
- Hard-boiled egg on 1 slice sprouted bread or 4 gluten-free crackers.
- ½–1 oz. 70 percent or higher cacao dark chocolate. Experiment with brands, because they don't all taste alike.
- 4 olives alone or combined with avocado slices or ½-1 oz. of hard cheese.
- 1 cup berries with 1–2 Tbsp. real, unsweetened whipped cream.
- Satisfying smoothie: 6 oz. plain, unsweetened yogurt; 1–3 Tbsp. whey vanilla protein, handful of berries, 1 tsp. of lime juice, and a touch of unsweetened vanilla almond milk.

## Smart Supplements

Trying to decide if in fact you need a nutritional supplement and then determining what products are safe and possibly beneficial can be overwhelming. Supplements are not permission for a reckless diet or lifestyle. They can, however, help you with your diet and lifestyle and support your body's natural functions, replenishing a deficiency and supporting metabolic pathways that enable key things to happen.

I'm going to swipe a broad stroke here and say that most people would benefit from the following four supplements, although there certainly are exceptions.

**Magnesium.** Magnesium is involved in many pathways in our body to regulate a wide variety of functions, including blood sugar, blood pressure, and bowel motility. The best form depends on your belly; magnesium citrate can help a constipated gut. Check with your physician before taking magnesium if your kidney function is compromised.

**Fish oils.** Fat is a sacred part of our cells and necessary for all cell function in all systems of our body, particularly cardiovascular and neuroendocrine. We've become fat-phobic and carb addicts, depleting ourselves of necessary essential fats, particularly EPA and DHA.

**Vitamin D.** Check your levels. Although vitamin D has received a lot of attention, questions still remain about its optimal blood levels and if we are even testing the correct vitamin D markers. But we do know that vitamin D receptors are found nearly from head to toe; in other words, it's involved in a lot of processes in our body. Also, a life lived indoors and then covered in sunblock when we are outdoors doesn't help us get our due vitamin D from its natural source: the sun.

**Coenzyme Q10.** CoQ10 or ubiquinone is an underutilized supplement in the United States with great cardiovascular benefit; the best cardiologists are aware of this. CoQ10 is integral for ATP production in the mitochondria of our cells and has great antioxidant capabilities in the cardiac cells. CoQ10 helps reduce the oxidized inflammatory form of LDL cholesterol. Aging and medications reduce our production of CoQ10, especially statin drugs. Anyone over forty but particularly those with cardiovascular risk and diabetes or on a statin drug would benefit from CoQ10. Research suggests the ubiquinol form is best absorbed.

# Appendix 4

## Resources

The following is a list of health-related websites, blogs, and YouTube videos.

## Organizations

Institute for Functional Medicine: www.functionalmedicine.org.

Dietitians in Integrative and Functional Medicine—For educational materials and finding a functional medicine dietitian: http://integrativerd.org.

American Academy of Nutrition and Dietetics—The website of registered dietitians; for education materials and finding a dietitian: www.eatright.org.

Environmental Working Group—Learn more about the toxins in our environment and how we can reduce our toxic load; publishes the "dirty dozen and clean fifteen" foods: www.ewg.org.

Consumer Lab—A great resource on the quality of herbal and dietary products: www.consumerlab.com.

Emerson Ecologics—Leading and trusted nutritional supplement distributor for health professionals, staffed by leading research physicians and naturopathic clinicians who study nutrition, health, and disease and the appropriate use of supplements. The companies for which Emerson distributes products are rated according to various standards of practice. Once on the website, click on "Emerson Quality Program" to learn about their high standard of products and their informative newsletters: http//www.emersonecologics.com.

The Hypertension Institute of Nashville—Mark Houston, MD; cardiologist and expert on the etiology and prevention of heart disease: http://www.hypertensioninstitute.com.

## Databases

CalorieKing—A wide database of nutrient content of most American foods: www.calorieking.com.

USDA—Nutrient list for foods: http://ndb.nal.usda.gov.

## Websites, Blogs, and Videos

Fruits & Veggies More Matters—Learn about the world of fruits and vegetables. There are a lot of foods to choose from: http://www.fruitsandveggiesmorematters.org.

University of Sydney's website on glycemic index: http://www.glycemicindex.com.

Monash University Medicine, Nursing and Health Sciences—Website on IBS and FODMAPs: http://www.med.monash.edu/cecs/gastro/fodmap/.

FODMAPs expert: www.Katescarlata.com.

Low-carb experts—Jeff Volek PhD, RD, and Stephen Phinney, MD, PhD. Two low-carb pioneers: http://www.artandscienceoflowcarb.com.

Cooking Light—Thousands of tested recipes in every category of food and flavor: www.cookinglight.com.

"The Bitter Truth" video on YouTube by Robert H. Lustig, MD (UCSF professor of pediatrics in the Division of Endocrinology). Sugar is sweet, but unfortunately it also has a bitter side: http://www.youtube.com/watch?v=oOWd5WMGAe4.

### Celiac or Gluten-Free Information

www.gfreeconnect.com.

www.celiac.com.

http://www.healthyvilli.org.

## Books

*The Art and Science of Low-Carbohydrate Eating* and *The Art and Science of Low-Carbohydrate Performance*, by Jeff Volk, RD, PhD, and Stephen Phinney, MD, PhD.

*The Great Cholesterol Myth*, by Stephen Sinatra, MD.

*Grain Brain*, by David Perlmutter, MD.

*Fat Chance*, by Robert Lustig, MD.

*Fat and Cholesterol Are GOOD* and *Ignore the Awkward*, both by Uffe Ravnskow.

*The Blood Sugar Solution*, by Mark Hyman, MD.

*The Diabetes Solution*, by Richard Bernstein, MD.

*Conquer Diabetes and Prediabetes: The Low-Carb Mediterranean Diet Plan*, by Steve Parker, MD.

*Breaking the Vicious Cycle: Intestinal Health through Diet*, by Elaine Gottschall.

*The New Atkins for a New You* by Eric Westman, MD, Stephen Phinney, MD, and Jeff Volek, PhD.

*The Inside Tract*, by Gerald Mullin, MD.

*Gut and Psychology Syndrome* (the GAPS diet), by Natasha Campbell-McBride, MD.

*The Paleo Diet for Athletes*, by Loren Cordain, PhD, and Joe Friel, MS.

*Wheat Belly*, by William Davis, MD.

*What Your Doctor May Not Tell You about Heart Disease*, by Mark Houston, MD.

*The Ultra Simple Diet*, by Mark Hyman, MD.

*The 21-Day Tummy Solution*, by Liz Vaccariello and Kate Scarlata, RD.

*Living Low Carb: Controlled Carbohydrate Eating for Long-Term Weight Loss*, by Jonny Bowden, PhD, CNS.

# References

Ahmadvand, H., H. Mabuchi, A. Nohara, J. Kobayahi, and M.A. Kawashiri. "Effects of Coenzyme Q(10) on LDL Oxidation in Vitro." Acta Medica Iranica 51.1 (2013): 12–18.

American Institute for Cancer Research (AICR)—ScienceNow: The Diabetes-Cancer Connection. Accessed August 2014.

American Psychiatric Association. "Substance-Related and Addictive Disorders DSM V." June 6, 2014. http://www.dsm5.org/Documents/Substance%20Use%20Disorder%20Fact%20Sheet.pdf.

Artemova, N. V., Z. M. Bumagina, A. S. Kasakov, V. V. Shubin, and B. Y. Gurvits. "Opioid Peptides Derived from Food Proteins Suppress Aggregation and Promote Reactivation of Partly Unfolded Stressed Proteins." Peptides 31.2 (2010): 332–38.

Astrup, A., J. Dyerberg, P. Elwood, K. Hermansen, F. B. Hu, M. U. Jakobsen, F. J. Kok, R. M. Krauss, J. M. Lecerf, P. Legrand, P. Nestel, U. Riserus, T. Sanders, A. Sinclair, S. Stender, T. Tholstrup, and W. C. Willett. "The Role of Reducing Intakes of Saturated Fat in the Prevention of Cardiovascular Disease: Where Does the Evidence Stand in 2010?" American Journal of Clinical Nutrition 93.4 (2011): 684–88.

Atkinson, W., S. Lockhart, P. Whorwell, B. Keevil, and L. Houghton. "Altered 5-Hydroxytryptamine Signaling in Patients with Constipation- and Diarrhea-Predominant Irritable Bowel Syndrome." Gastroenterology 130.1 (2006): 34–43.

Azad, M. B., T. Konya, H. Maughan, D. S. Guttman, C. J. Field, R. S. Chari, M. R. Sears, A. B. Becker, J. A. Scott, and A. L. Kozyrskyj. "Gut Microbiota of Healthy Canadian Infants: Profiles by Mode of Delivery and Infant Diet at 4 Months." Canadian Medical Association Journal 185.5 (2013): 385–94.

Barrett, J. S., and P. R. Gibson. "Fermentable Oligosaccharides, Disaccharides, Monosaccharides and Polyols (FODMAPs) and Nonallergic Food Intolerance: FODMAPs or Food Chemicals?" Therapeutic Advances in Gastroenterology 5.4 (2012): 261–68.

Barrett, J. S. "Probiotic Effects on Intestinal Fermentation Patterns in Patients with Irritable Bowel Syndrome." *World Journal of Gastroenterology* 14.32 (2008): 5020.

Barrett, J. S., P. M. Irving, S. J. Shepherd, J. G. Muir, and P. R. Gibson. "Comparison of the Prevalence of Fructose and Lactose Malabsorption across Chronic Intestinal Disorders." *Alimentary Pharmacology & Therapeutics* 30.2 (2009): 165–74.

Bernstein, R. K. *Dr. Bernstein's Diabetes Solution: The Complete Guide to Achieving Normal Blood Sugars.* New York: Little, Brown, 2007.

Bessesen, D. H. "Effect of a Low-Carbohydrate Diet on Appetite, Blood Glucose Levels, and Insulin Resistance in Obese Patients with Type 2 Diabetes." *Yearbook of Endocrinology* (2006): 149–51.

Biesiekierski, J. R., O. Rosella, R. Rose, K. Liels, J. S. Barrett, S. J. Shepherd, P. R. Gibson, and J. G. Muir. "Quantification of Fructans, Galacto-oligosaccharides, and Other Short-Chain Carbohydrates in Processed Grains and Cereals." *Journal of Human Nutrition and Dietetics* 24.2 (2011): 154–76.

Block, G., C. Jensen, T. Dalvi, E. Norkus, M. Hudes, P. Crawford, N. Holland, E. Fung, L. Schumacher, and P. Harmatz. "Vitamin C Treatment Reduces Elevated C-Reactive Protein." *Free Radical Biology and Medicine* 46.1 (2009): 70–77.

Bowden, J., and S. T. Sinatra. *The Great Cholesterol Myth: Why Lowering Your Cholesterol Won't Prevent Heart Disease—and the Statin-Free Plan That Will.* Beverly, MA: Fair Winds, 2012.

Brinkworth, G. D., M. Noakes, P. M. Clifton, and A. R. Bird. "Comparative Effects of Very Low-Carbohydrate, High-Fat and High-Carbohydrate, Low-Fat Weight-Loss Diets on Bowel Habit and Faecal Short-Chain Fatty Acids and Bacterial Populations." *British Journal of Nutrition* 101.10 (2009): 1493.

Buyken, A. E., V. Flood, M. Empson, E. Rochtchina, A. W. Barclay, J. Brand-Miller, and P. Mitchell. "Carbohydrate Nutrition and Inflammatory Disease Mortality in Older Adults." *American Journal of Clinical Nutrition* 92.3 (2010): 634–43.

CalorieKing. *Calorie Counter—Calories in Sugar.* http://www.calorieking.com/calories-in-sugar.html. Accessed June 10, 2014.

Campbell-McBride, N. *Gut and Psychology Syndrome: Natural Treat-*

*ment for Autism, Dyspraxia, A.D.D., Dyslexia, A.D.H.D., Depression, Schizophrenia.* Cambridge, UK: Medinform Pub., 2010.

Canny, G. O., and B. A. Mccormick. "Bacteria in the Intestine: Helpful Residents or Enemies from Within?" Infection and Immunity 76.8 (2008): 3360–373.

"Carbohydrate Counting and Exchange Lists." United States Department of Agriculture. http://fnic.nal.usda.gov/diet-and-disease/diabetes/carbohydrate-counting-and-exchange-lists. Accessed July 22, 2014.

Carroll, C. H. "Protein and Exercise." In Sports Nutrition: A Guide for the Professional Working with Active People. Chicago, Illinois: American Dietetic Association, 2000. 33–50.

Center for Substance Abuse Treatment, "DM IV TR Criteria for Substance Dependence." *Appendix C DSM-IV-TR Material.* U.S. National Library of Medicine, April 18, 0000. http://www.ncbi.nlm.nih.gov/books/NBK64247/. Accessed July 8, 2014.

Chatham, J. C. "Lactate—the Forgotten Fuel!" *Journal of Physiology* 542.2 (2002): 333.

Choi, S.-W., and S. Friso. "Epigenetics: A New Bridge between Nutrition and Health." *Advances in Nutrition: An International Review Journal* 1.1 (2010): 8–16.

"ChooseMyPlate.gov." http://www.choosemyplate.gov/. Accessed July 10, 2014.

"Clinical and Laboratory Characteristics of Diabetic Ketoacidosis in Adult Diabetic Patients." *Internet Journal of Endocrinology* 3.2 (2007).

Colorado State University, "Functional Anatomy of the Endocrine Pancreas.", (2006): http://arbl.cvmbs.colostate.edu/hbooks/pathphys/endocrine/pancreas/anatomy.Accessed June 2014.

Conlee, R. K., R. M. Lawler, and P. E. Ross. "Effects of Glucose or Fructose Feeding on Glycogen Repletion in Muscle and Liver after Exercise or Fasting." *Annals of Nutrition and Metabolism* 31.2 (1987): 126–32.

Cordain, L., and J. Friel. *The Paleo Diet for Athletes: The Ancient Nutritional Formula for Peak Athletic Performance.* New York: Rodale, 2012.

"Coronary Heart Disease Death, Nonfatal Acute Myocardial Infarction, and Other Clinical Outcomes in the Multiple Risk Factor Intervention Trial." *American Journal of Cardiology* 58.1 (1986): 1–13.

Craft, S. "Insulin Resistance and Alzheimer's Disease Pathogenesis: Potential Mechanisms and Implications for Treatment." *Current Alzheimer's Research* 4.2 (2007): 147–52.

"A Critique of Low-Carbohydrate Ketogenic Weight Reduction Regimens: A Review of Dr. Atkins' Diet Revolution." *JAMA: The Journal of the American Medical Association* 224.10 (1973): 1415–19.

Dalmasso, G., F. Cottrez, V. Imbert, P. Lagadec, J.-F. Peyron, P. Rampal, D. Czerucka, and H. Groux. "Saccharomyces Boulardii Inhibits Inflammatory Bowel Disease by Trapping T Cells in Mesenteric Lymph Nodes." *Gastroenterology* 131.6 (2006): 1812–25.

Dandona, P. "Metabolic Syndrome: A Comprehensive Perspective Based on Interactions between Obesity, Diabetes, and Inflammation." *Circulation* 111.11 (2005): 1448–54.

Davis, W. *Wheat Belly: Lose the Wheat, Lose the Weight, and Find Your Path Back to Health.* Emmaus, PA: Rodale, 2011.

De Groot, M. J. M. *The Effect of Lactate on the Normoxic, Ischemic and Reperfused Heart.* University Library, Maastricht University [Host], Maastricht, The Netherlands,1992.

"Diabetes Mellitus, Fasting Glucose, and Risk of Cause-Specific Death." The Emerging Risk Factors Collaboration: Seshasai, RK, Kaptoge, S., Thompson, A. et al. New England Journal of Medicine 364.9 (2011): 829–41.

"Dietary Reference Intakes for Macronutrients Tables." United States Department of Agriculture. http://fnic.nal.usda.gov/dietary-guidance/dietary-reference-intakes/dri-tables. Accessed June 6, 2014.

Duncan, S. H., A. Belenguer, G. Holtrop, A. M. Johnstone, H. J. Flint, and G. E. Lobley. "Reduced Dietary Intake of Carbohydrates by Obese Subjects Results in Decreased Concentrations of Butyrate and Butyrate-Producing Bacteria in Feces." *Applied and Environmental Microbiology* 73.4 (2007): 1073–78.

Englyst, K. N., and H. N. Englyst. "Carbohydrate Bioavailability." *British Journal of Nutrition* 94.01 (2005): 1.

Erbach, M., H. Mehnert, and O. Schnell. "Diabetes and the Risk for Colorectal Cancer." *Journal of Diabetes and Its Complications* 26.1 (2012): 50–55.

Esposito, K. "Effect of a Mediterranean-Style Diet on Endothelial Dysfunction and Markers of Vascular Inflammation in the Metabolic Syndrome: A Randomized Trial." *JAMA: The Journal of the American Medical Association* 292.12 (2004): 1440–46.

Evans, D. F., G. Pye, R. Bramley, A. G. Clark, T. J. Dyson, and J. D. Hardcastle. "Measurement of Gastrointestinal pH Profiles in Normal Ambulant Human Subjects." *Gut* 29.8 (1988): 1035–41.

Falchi, M., J. S. El-Sayed Moustafa, P. Takousis, F. Pesce, A. Bonnefond, J. C. Andersson-Assarsson, P. H. Sudmant, R. Dorajoo, M. N. Al-Shafai, L. Bottolo, E. Ozdemir, H.-C. So, R. W. Davies, A. Patrice, R. Dent, M. Mangino, P. G. Hysi, A. Dechaume, M. Huyvaert, J. Skinner, M. Pigeyre, R. Caiazzo, V. Raverdy, E. Vaillant, S. Field, B. Balkau, M. Marre, S. Visvikis-Siest, J. Weill, O. Poulain-Godefroy, P. Jacobson, L. Sjostrom, C. J. Hammond, P. Deloukas, P. C. Sham, R. McPherson, J. Lee, E. S. Tai, R. Sladek, L. M. S. Carlsson, A. Walley, E. E. Eichler, F. Pattou, T. D. Spector, and P. Froguel. "Low Copy Number of the Salivary Amylase Gene Predisposes to Obesity." Nature Genetics 46 (2014): 492-497.

Fasano, A. "Physiological, Pathological, and Therapeutic Implications of Zonulin-Mediated Intestinal Barrier Modulation." *American Journal of Pathology* 173.5 (2008): 1243–52.

Fasano, A. "Zonulin and Its Regulation of Intestinal Barrier Function: The Biological Door to Inflammation, Autoimmunity, and Cancer." *Physiological Reviews* 91.1 (2011): 151–75.

Feinman, R. D., and J. S. Volek. "Carbohydrate Restriction as the Default Treatment for Type 2 Diabetes and Metabolic Syndrome." *Scandinavian Cardiovascular Journal* 42.4 (2008): 256–63.

Flood, A., L. Strayer, C. Schairer, and A. Schatzkin. "Diabetes and Risk of Incident Colorectal Cancer in a Prospective Cohort of Women." *Cancer Causes & Control* 21.8 (2010): 1277–84.

Ford, R., and P. Kinvig. "The Gluten Syndrome: A Neurological Disease." *Medical Hypotheses* 73.3 (2009): 438–40.

Forsythe, C. E., S. D. Phinney, R. D. Feinman, B. M. Volk, D. Freidenreich, E. Quann, K. Ballard, M. J. Puglisi, C. M. Maresh, W. J. Kraemer, D. M. Bibus, M. L. Fernandez, and J. S. Volek. "Limited Effect of Dietary Saturated Fat on Plasma Saturated Fat in the Context of a Low Carbohydrate Diet." *Lipids* 45.10 (2010): 947–62.

Forsythe, C. E., S. D. Phinney, M. L. Fernandez, E. E. Quann, R. J. Wood, D. M. Bibus, W. J. Kraemer, R. D. Feinman, and J. S. Volek. "Comparison of Low Fat and Low Carbohydrate Diets on Circulating Fatty Acid Composition and Markers of Inflammation." *Lipids* 43.1 (2008): 65–77.

Frassetto, L. A., M. Schloetter, M. Mietus-Synder, R. C. Morris, and A. Sebastian. "Metabolic and Physiologic Improvements from Consuming a Paleolithic, Hunter-Gatherer Type Diet." *European Journal of Clinical Nutrition* 63.8 (2009): 947–55.

Freedland, S. J., and W. J. Aronson. "Re: Weight Loss with a Low-Carbohydrate, Mediterranean, or Low-Fat Diet." *European Urology* 55.1 (2009): 249–50.

Fukudome Sl,, Yoshikawa M. "Opioid Peptides Derived from Wheat Gluten: Their Isolation and Characterization." FEBS Lett. 296.1 (1992):107-11.Accessed August 9, 2014.

Gagné, L. "The Glycemic Index and Glycemic Load in Clinical Practice." *EXPLORE: The Journal of Science and Healing* 4.1 (2008): 66–69.

Gardner, C. D., et al. "Insulin Resistance—An Effect Moderator of Weight Loss Success on High vs. Low Carbohydrate Diets." *Obesity* 16 (2008): S82.

Ghoshal, U. C. "How to Interpret Hydrogen Breath Tests." *Journal of Neurogastroenterology and Motility* 17.3 (2011): 312.

Gill, S. R. "Metagenomic Analysis of the Human Distal Gut Microbiome." *Science* 312.5778 (2006): 1355–59.

Grabitske, H. A., and J. L. Slavin. "Gastrointestinal Effects of Low-Digestible Carbohydrates." *Critical Reviews in Food Science and Nutrition* 49.4 (2009): 327–60.

Grabitske, H. A., and J. L. Slavin. "Low-Digestible Carbohydrates in Practice." *Journal of the American Dietetic Association* 108.10 (2008): 1677–81.

Grassi, D., G. Desideri, S. Necozione, C. Lippi, A. Mazza, G. Croce, L. Valeri, A. Garofalo, G. Properzi, J. Blumberg, and C. Ferri. "Flavanol-Rich Dark Chocolate Decreases Blood Pressure, Improves Endothelium-Dependent Vasorelaxation, and Ameliorates Insulin Sensitivity in Patients with Essential Hypertension." *High Blood Pressure & Cardiovascular Prevention* 12.3 (2005): 185.

Haast, R. A., and A. J. Kiliaan. "Impact of Fatty Acids on Brain Circulation, Structure, and Function." *Prostaglandins, Leukotrienes and Essential Fatty Acids (PLEFA)* (2014).

Habba, S. F. "Diarrhea Predominant Irritable Bowel Syndrome (IBS-D): Fact or Fiction." *Medical Hypotheses* 76.1 (2011): 97–99.

Hays, James H. "The Hunter-Gatherer Diet." *Mayo Clinic Proceedings* 79.5 (2004): 703.

Heilbronn, L. K. "Effect of 6-Month Calorie Restriction on Biomarkers of Longevity, Metabolic Adaptation, and Oxidative Stress in Overweight Individuals: A Randomized Controlled Trial." *JAMA: The Journal of the American Medical Association* 295.13 (2006): 1539–48.

Hininger, I., M. Chopra, D. I. Thurnham, F. Laporte, M.-J. Richard, A. Favier, and A.-M. Roussel. "Effect of Increased Fruit and Vegetable Intake on the Susceptibility of Lipoprotein to Oxidation in Smokers." *European Journal of Clinical Nutrition* 51.9 (1997): 601–6.

Hitman, G. A. "Diabetic Ketoacidosis: Could We Do Better?" *Diabetic Medicine* 30.5 (2013): 511.

Ho, V. W., K. Leung, A. Hsu, B. Luk, J. Lai, S. Y. Shen, A. I. Minchinton, D. Waterhouse, M. B. Bally, W. Lin, B. H. Nelson, L. M. Sly, and G. Krystal. "A Low-Carbohydrate, High-Protein Diet Slows Tumor Growth and Prevents Cancer Initiation." *Cancer Research* 71.13 (2011): 4484–93.

Hotoleanu, C. "Genetic Determination of Irritable Bowel Syndrome." *World Journal of Gastroenterology* 14.43 (2008): 6636.

Houston, M. C. *Handbook of Hypertension.* Chichester, UK: Wiley-Blackwell, 2009.

Houston, M. C. *What Your Doctor May Not Tell You about Heart Disease.* New York: Grand Central Life & Style, 2012.

Howard, B. V. "Low-Fat Dietary Pattern and Risk of Cardiovascular Disease: The Women's Health Initiative Randomized Controlled Dietary Modification Trial." *JAMA: The Journal of the American Medical Association* 295.6 (2006): 655–66.

Hu, F. B., J. B. Meigs, T. Y. Li, N. Rifai, and J. E. Manson. "Inflammatory Markers and Risk of Developing Type 2 Diabetes in Women." *Diabetes* 53.3 (2004): 693–700.

Hyde, M. J., and N. Modi. "The Long-Term Effects of Birth by Caesarean Section: The Case for a Randomised Controlled Trial." *Early Human Development* 88.12 (2012): 943–49.

Hyman, M. *The Blood Sugar Solution: The Ultrahealthy Program for Losing Weight, Preventing Disease, and Feeling Great Now!* New York: Little, Brown, 2012.

Gardner, CD, Kiazand, A, Alhassan, S, Kim S, Stafford RS, Balise RR, Kraemer, HC, King, AC. Comparison of the Atkins, Zone, Ornish, and LEARN Diets for Change in Weight and Related Risk Factors among Overweight Premenopausal Women: The A to Z Weight Loss Study: A Randomized Trial." JAMA: The Journal of the American Medical Association 298.2 (2007): 178.

Jabekk, P. T., I. A. Moe, H. D. Meen, S. E. Tomten, and A. T. Høstmark. "Resistance Training in Overweight Women on a Ketogenic Diet Conserved Lean Body Mass While Reducing Body Fat." *Nutrition & Metabolism* 7.1 (2010): 17.

Jakobsen, M. U., E. J. O'Reilly, B. L. Heitmann, M. A. Pereira, K. Balter, G. E. Fraser, U. Goldbourt, G. Hallmans, P. Knekt, S. Liu, P. Pietinen, D. Spiegelman, J. Stevens, J. Virtamo, W. C. Willett, and A. Ascherio. "Major Types of Dietary Fat and Risk of Coronary Heart Disease: A Pooled Analysis of 11 Cohort Studies." *American Journal of Clinical Nutrition* 89.5 (2009): 1425–32.

Jarzab, A., J. Stopyra, and K. Fyderek. "The Role of Small Intestinal Bacterial Overgrowth in the Pathogenesis of Gastroesophageal Reflux." *Gastroenterology* 124.4 (2003): A411.

Johansen, K. L. "Increased Diabetes Mellitus Risk with Statin Use: Comment on 'Statin Use and Risk of Diabetes Mellitus in Postmenopausal Women in the Women's Health Initiative.'" *Archives of Internal Medicine* 172.2 (2012): 152.

Jones, D. S. *Textbook of Functional Medicine*. Gig Harbor, WA: Institute for Functional Medicine, 2010.

Kalman, B., and T. H. Brannagan. "Neurological Manifestations of Gluten Sensitivity." In *Neuroimmunology in Clinical Practice*. Malden, MA: Blackwell, 2008.

Kang, J. X. "The Coming of Age of Nutrigenetics and Nutrigenomics." *Journal of Nutrigenetics and Nutrigenomics* 5.1 (2012): 1-11..

Key, T. J., and E. A. Spencer. "Carbohydrates and Cancer: An Overview of the Epidemiological Evidence." *European Journal of Clinical Nutrition* 61 (2007): S112–S121.

Kim, J.-A. "Reciprocal Relationships between Insulin Resistance and Endothelial Dysfunction: Molecular and Pathophysiological Mechanisms." *Circulation* 113.15 (2006): 1888–904.

Klement, R. J., and U. Kämmerer. "Is There a Role for Carbohydrate Restriction in the Treatment and Prevention of Cancer?" *Nutrition & Metabolism* 8.1 (2011): 75.

Lachance, L. R., and K. McKenzie. "Biomarkers of Gluten Sensitivity in Patients with Non-affective Psychosis: A Meta-analysis." *Schizophrenia Research* 152.2–3 (2014): 521–27.

Lagiou, P., S. Sandin, E. Weiderpass, A. Lagiou, L. Mucci, D. Trichopoulos, and H.-O. Adami. "Low Carbohydrate/High Protein Diet and Mortality in a Cohort of Swedish Women." *Journal of Internal Medicine* 261.4 (2007): 366–74.

Larsson, S. C. E., L. Bergkuist, and A. Wolk. "High-fat Dairy Food and Conjugated Linoleic Acid Intakes in Relation to Colorectal Cancer Incidence in the Swedish Mammography Cohort 1,2,3." *American Journal of Clinical Nutrition* 82.4 (2005): 894–900.

Layman, L. K., et al. "Dietary Protein and Exercise Have Additive Effects on Body Composition during Weight Loss in Adult Women." *Journal of Nutrition* 135.8 (2005): 1903–10.

Leibenluft, E., P. L. Fiero, J. J. Bartko, D. E. Moul, and N. E. Rosenthal. "Depressive Symptoms and the Self-Reported Use of Alcohol, Caffeine, and Carbohydrates in Normal Volunteers and Four Groups of Psychiatric Outpatients." *Journal of Addictions Nursing* 6.1 (1994): 32–41.

Lembo, A. J., B. Neri, J. Tolley, D. Barken, S. Carroll, and H. Pan. "Use of Serum Biomarkers in a Diagnostic Test for Irritable

Bowel Syndrome." *Alimentary Pharmacology & Therapeutics* 29.8 (2009): 834–42.

Lin, H. C. "Small Intestinal Bacterial Overgrowth: A Framework for Understanding Irritable Bowel Syndrome." *JAMA: The Journal of the American Medical Association* 292.7 (2004): 852–58.

Lindegren, C. C., and G. Lindegren. "Proximity of Genes Controlling the Fermentation of Similar Carbohydrates in Saccharomyces." *Nature* 170.4336 (1952): 965–68.

"The Lipid Research Clinics Coronary Primary Prevention Trial. Results of 6 Years of Post-trial Follow-up. The Lipid Research Clinics Investigators." *Archives of Internal Medicine* 152.7 (1992): 1399–410.

Lord, RS, and JA Brailey. "Clinical Applications of Urinary Organic Acids. Part 2. Dysbiosis Markers." *Alternative Medicine Review* 4 (2008): 292-306.

"Low Carb Diet Program and Weight Loss Plan | Atkins." Online: www.atkins.com  a.

Lustig, R. H. *Fat Chance: Beating the Odds against Sugar, Processed Food, Obesity, and Disease.* New York, Hudson Street Press, 2012.

Lustig, R. H., L. A. Schmidt, and C. D. Brindis. "Public Health: The Toxic Truth about Sugar." *Nature* 482.7383 (2012): 27–29.

Macfarlane, S. "Microbial Biofilm Communities in the Gastrointestinal Tract." *Journal of Clinical Gastroenterology* 42 (2008): S142–S143.

McOrist, A. L., R. B. Miller, A. R. Bird, J. B. Keogh, M. Noakes, D. L. Topping, and M. A. Conlon. "Fecal Butyrate Levels Vary Widely among Individuals but Are Usually Increased by a Diet High in Resistant Starch." *Journal of Nutrition* 141.5 (2011): 883–89.

Moreno-Navarrete, J. M., M. Sabater, F. Ortega, W. Ricart, and J. M. Fernández-Real. "Circulating Zonulin, a Marker of Intestinal Permeability, Is Increased in Association with Obesity-Associated Insulin Resistance." Ed. Massimo Federici. *PLoS ONE* 7.5 (2012): E37160.

Mullin, G. E. "Article Commentary: High-Fat Diet Determines the Composition of the Murine Gut Microbiome Independently of Obesity." *Nutrition in Clinical Practice* 25.3 (2010): 310–11.

Mullin, G. E., and K. M. Swift. *The Inside Tract: Your Good Gut Guide to Great Digestive Health.* New York: Rodale, 2011.

Muraki, M., Y. Fujiwara, H. Machida, H. Okazaki, M. Sogawa, H. Yamagami, T. Tanigawa, M. Shiba, K. Watanabe, K. Tominaga, T. Watanabe, and T. Arakawa. "Role of Small Intestinal Bacterial Overgrowth in Severe Small Intestinal Damage in Chronic Non-steroidal Anti-inflammatory Drug Users." *Scandinavian Journal of Gastroenterology* (2014): 1–7.

Murray, J. A., S. B. Moore, C. T. Van Dyke, B. D. Lahr, R. A. Dierkhising, A. R. Zinsmeister, L. J. Melton, C. M. Kroning, M. El–Yousseff, and A. J. Czaja. "HLA DQ Gene Dosage and Risk and Severity of Celiac Disease." *Clinical Gastroenterology and Hepatology* 5.12 (2007): 1406–12.

"New IBS & CIC Monograph." http://www.acg.gi.org/. Accessed April 5, 2014.

Nordmoe, E. D. "Kiss High Blood Pressure Goodbye: The Relationship between Dark Chocolate and Hypertension." *Teaching Statistics* 30.2 (2008): 34–38.

O'Keefe, J. H., and L. Cordain. "Cardiovascular Disease Resulting from a Diet and Lifestyle at Odds with Our Paleolithic Genome: How to Become a 21st-Century Hunter-Gatherer." *Mayo Clinic Proceedings* 79.1 (2004): 101–8.

Olmstead, Stephen F. "Life on the Edge: The Clinical Implications of Gastrointestinal Biofilm." Online: *Free Online Library.* http://www.multibriefs.com/briefs/icim/biofilm.pdfAccessed   August 10, 2014.

Ong, D. K., S. B. Mitchell, J. S. Barrett, S. J. S., P. M. Irving, J. R. Biesiekierski, S. Smith, P. R. Gibson, and J. G. Muir. "Manipulation of Dietary Short-Chain Carbohydrates Alters the Pattern of Gas Production and Genesis of Symptoms in Irritable Bowel Syndrome." *Journal of Gastroenterology and Hepatology* 25.8 (2010): 1366–73.

Otero, M. "Towards a Pro-inflammatory and Immunomodulatory Emerging Role of Leptin." *Rheumatology* 45.8 (2006): 944–50.

Pagana, K. D., and T. J. Pagana. *Mosby's Manual of Diagnostic and Laboratory Tests.* St. Louis: Mosby/Elsevier, 2010.

Palmer, W. K. "Hormonal Regulation of Myocardial Lipolysis." *Medicine & Science in Sports & Exercise* 15.4 (1983): 331-5.

Parker, S. *Conquering Diabetes and Pre-diabetes; The Low-Carb Mediterranean Diet Plan.* pxHealth; Scottsdale, Arizona.First edition (2011).

Perlmutter, D., and K. Loberg. *Grain Brain: The Surprising Truth about Wheat, Carbs, and Sugar—Your Brain's Silent Killers.* Little, Brown and Company, New York, 2013.

Perry, G. H., N. J. Dominy, K. G. Claw, A. S. Lee, H. Fiegler, R. Redon, J. Werner, F. A. Villanea, J. L. Mountain, R. Misra, N. P. Carter, C. Lee, and A. C. Stone. "Diet and the Evolution of Human Amylase Gene Copy Number Variation." *Nature Genetics* 39.10 (2007): 1256–60.

Phinney, S. D., B. R. Bistrian, R. R. Wolfe, and G. L. Blackburn. "The Human Metabolic Response to Chronic Ketosis without Caloric Restriction: Physical and Biochemical Adaptation." *Metabolism* 32.8 (1983): 757–68.

Phinney, S. D., B. R. Bistrian, W. J. Evans, E. Gervino, and G. L. Blackburn. "The Human Metabolic Response to Chronic Ketosis without Caloric Restriction: Preservation of Submaximal Exercise Capability with Reduced Carbohydrate Oxidation." *Metabolism* 32.8 (1983): 769–76.

Phinney, S. D., E. S. Horton, J. S. Hanson, E. Danforth, and B. M. Lagrange. "Capacity for Moderate Exercise in Obese Subjects after Adaptation to a Hypocaloric, Ketogenic Diet." *Journal of Clinical Investigation* 66.5 (1980): 1152–61.

Pietrucha, T. "The Genetics of Metabolic Syndrome." *Medical Science and Technology* 54 (2013): 48–53.

Pimentel, M., et al. "Lower Frequency of MMC Is Found in IBS Subjects with Abnormal Lactulose Breath Test, Suggesting Bacterial Overgrowth." Digestive Diseases and Sciences. 47 (2002): 2639–43.

Pimentel, M., Y. Kong, and S. Park. "IBS Subjects with Methane on Lactulose Breath Test Have Lower Postprandial Serotonin Levels Than Subjects with Hydrogen." *Digestive Diseases and Sciences* 49.1 (2004): 84–87.

Pool-Zobel, B. L. "Inulin-type Fructans and Reduction in Colon Cancer Risk: Review of Experimental and Human Data." *British Journal of Nutrition* 93.S1 (2005): S73.

Pradhan, A. D. "C-Reactive Protein, Interleukin 6, and Risk of Developing Type 2 Diabetes Mellitus." *JAMA: The Journal of the American Medical Association* 286.3 (2001): 327–34.

Quigley, E. M. M. "Small Intestinal Bacterial Overgrowth." *Current Opinion in Gastroenterology* (2014): 1.

Rauchenzauner, M., J. Klepper, B. Leiendecker, G. Luef, K. Rostasy, and C. Ebenbichler. "Effects of Long-term Ketogenic Diet on Glucose Metabolism, Lipid Profile, and Adipocytokines in Epileptic Children with Glut1 Deficiency Syndrome." Neuropediatrics 39.01 (2008).

Ravnskov, U. *Ignore the Awkward!: How the Cholesterol Myths Are Kept Alive.* Charleston, SC: CreateSpace, 2010.

Ravnskov, U., and J. M. Kauffman. Fat and Cholesterol Are Good for You. GB Publishing, Sweden, 2009.

Reddymasu, S. C., and R. W. McCallum. "Small Intestinal Bacterial Overgrowth in Gastroparesis." *Journal of Clinical Gastroenterology* 44.1 (2010): E8–E13.

Reddymasu, S. C., S. Sostarich, and R. W. McCallum. "Small Intestinal Bacterial Overgrowth in Irritable Bowel Syndrome: Are There Any Predictors?" *BMC Gastroenterology* 10.1 (2010): 23.

Renz-Polster, H., M. R. David, A. S. Buist, W. M. Vollmer, E. A. O'Connor, E. A. Frazier, and M. A. Wall. "Caesarean Section Delivery and the Risk of Allergic Disorders in Childhood." *Clinical Experimental Allergy* 35.11 (2005): 1466–72.

"Retraction: Periodontitis and Cardiovascular Disease: Floss and Reduce a Potential Risk Factor for CVD." *Angiology* 62.1 (2010): 62–67.

Ridker, P. M., R. J. Glynn, and C. H. Hennekens. "C-Reactive Protein Adds to the Predictive Value of Total and HDL Cholesterol in Determining Risk of First Myocardial Infarction." *Circulation* 97.20 (1998): 2007–11.

Roberts, R. O., et al. "Relative Intake of Macronutrients Impacts Risk of Mild Cognitive Impairment or Dementia." *Journal of Alzheimer's Disease* 32.2 (2012): 329–39.

Rosenbloom, C. "Protein and Exercise." In *Sports Nutrition: A Guide for the Professional Working with Active People*. Chicago: American Dietetic Association, 2000. 33–50.

Sapone, A. "Zonulin Upregulation Is Associated with Increased Gut Permeability in Subjects with Type 1 Diabetes and Their Relatives." *Diabetes* 55.5 (2006): 1443–49.

Scarlata, K. "Irritable Bowel Syndrome: FODMAPs, Fat, Fiber and Flora.", Wolf Rinke Associates, Inc. Clarksville, MD. (2012).

Shai, I., D. Schwarzfuchs, Y. Henkin, D. R. Shahar, S. Witkow, I. Greenberg, R. Golan, D. Fraser, A. Bolotin, H. Vardi, O. Tangi-Rozental, R. Zuk-Ramot, B. Sarusi, D. Brickner, Z. Schwartz, E. Sheiner, R. Marko, E. Katorza, J. Thiery, G. M. Fiedler, M. Blüher, M. Stumvoll, and M. J. Stampfer. "Weight Loss with a Low-Carbohydrate, Mediterranean, or Low-Fat Diet." *New England Journal of Medicine* 359.3 (2008): 229–41.

Shils, M. E., and M. Shike. *Modern Nutrition in Health and Disease*. Philadelphia: Lippincott Williams & Wilkins, 2006.

Shukitt-Hale, B. "Blueberries and Neuronal Aging." *Gerontology* 58.6 (2012): 518–23.

Simopoulos, A. "Dietary Omega-3 Fatty Acid Deficiency and High Fructose Intake in the Development of Metabolic Syndrome Brain, Metabolic Abnormalities, and Non-Alcoholic Fatty Liver Disease." *Nutrients* 5.8 (2013): 2901–23.

Simren, M. "Use and Abuse of Hydrogen Breath Tests." *Gut* 55.3 (2006): 297-303.

Sokhanenkova, N. Y, L. S. Asmakova, V. A. Dubinin, J. D. Bespalova, and A. A. Kamensky. "Neurotropic Effects of Some Exorphins—Natural Exogenous Opioid Peptides." *Biological Psychiatry* 42.1 (1997): 48S.

Song, S. J., M. G. Dominguez-Bello, and R. Knight. "How Delivery Mode and Feeding Can Shape the Bacterial Community in the Infant Gut." *Canadian Medical Association Journal* 185.5 (2013): 373–74.

Sonksen, P. "Insulin: Understanding Its Action in Health and Disease." *British Journal of Anaesthesia* 85.1 (2000): 69–79.

Spreadbury, I. "Comparison with Ancestral Diets Suggest Dense

Acellular Carbohydrates Promote an Inflammatory Microbiota and May Be the Primary Dietary Cause of Leptin Resistance and Obesity." *Journal of Diabetes, Metabolic Syndrome and Obesity* 5 (2012): 175–89.

Stafstrom, C. E., and J. M. Rho. "The Ketogenic Diet as a Treatment Paradigm for Diverse Neurological Disorders." *Frontiers in Pharmacology* 3 (2012). http://www.ncbi.nlm.nih.gov/pmc/articles/PMC3321471/

Staudacher, H. M., M. C. E. Lomer, J. L. Anderson, J. S. Barrett, J. G. Muir, P. M. Irving, and K. Whelan. "Fermentable Carbohydrate Restriction Reduces Luminal Bifidobacteria and Gastrointestinal Symptoms in Patients with Irritable Bowel Syndrome." *Journal of Nutrition* 142.8 (2012): 1510–18.

Staudacher, H. M., K. Whelan, P. M. Irving, and M. C. E. Lomer. "Comparison of Symptom Response Following Advice for a Diet Low in Fermentable Carbohydrates (FODMAPs) versus Standard Dietary Advice in Patients with Irritable Bowel Syndrome." *Journal of Human Nutrition and Dietetics* 24.5 (2011): 487–95.

Steen, Eric, et al. "Impaired Insulin and Insulin-Like Growth Factor Expression and Signaling Mechanisms in Alzheimer's Disease—Is This Type 3 Diabetes?" Journal of Alzheimer's Disease 7.1 (2005): 63–80.

Suh, S., and K.-W. Kim. "Diabetes and Cancer: Is Diabetes Causally Related to Cancer?" *Diabetes & Metabolism Journal* 35.3 (2011): 193.

Tana, C., Y. Umesaki, A. Imaoka, T. Handa, M. Kanazawa, and S. Fukudo. "Altered Profiles of Intestinal Microbiota and Organic Acids May Be the Origin of Symptoms in Irritable Bowel Syndrome." Neurogastroenterology & Motility (2009).

Tilg, H., and A. Kaser. "Gut Microbiome, Obesity, and Metabolic Dysfunction." *Journal of Clinical Investigation* 121.6 (2011): 2126–32.

Tirosh A1, Shai I, Tekes-Manova D, Israeli E, Pereg D, Shochat T, Kochba I, Rudich A; Israeli Diabetes Research Group. "Normal Fasting Plasma Glucose Levels and Type 2 Diabetes in Young Men." New England Journal of Medicine 354.22 (2006): 2401.

Trichopoulou, A., T. Psaltopoulou, P. Orfanos, C.-C. Hsieh, and

D. Trichopoulos. "Low-Carbohydrate–High-Protein Diet and Long-Term Survival in a General Population Cohort." *European Journal of Clinical Nutrition* 61.5 (2007): 575-81.

Turnbaugh, P. J., and J. I. Gordon. "The Core Gut Microbiome, Energy Balance, and Obesity." *Journal of Physiology* 587.17 (2009): 4153–58.

University of Sydney 2011. www.glycemicindex.com.

Usai, P., A. Serra, B. Marini, S. Mariotti, L. Satta, M. Boi, A. Spanu, G. Loi, and M. Piga. "Frontal Cortical Perfusion Abnormalities Related to Gluten Intake and Associated Autoimmune Disease in Adult Coeliac Disease: 99mTc-ECD Brain SPECT Study." *Digestive and Liver Disease* 36.8 (2004): 513–18.

U.S. Department of Agriculture and U.S. Department of Health and Human Services. "Dietary Guidelines for Americans, Washington, DC (2010): 7th edition

Vander Heiden, M. G., L. C. Cantley, and C. B. Thompson. "Understanding the Warburg Effect: The Metabolic Requirements of Cell Proliferation." *Science* 324.5930 (2009): 1029–33.

Visser, J., J. Rozing, A. Sapone, K. Lammers, and A. Fasano. "Tight Junctions, Intestinal Permeability, and Autoimmunity." *Annals of the New York Academy of Sciences* 1165.1 (2009): 195–205.

Volek, J. S. "Carbohydrate Restriction Uniquely Benefits Metabolic Syndrome and Saturated Fat Metabolism." *BMC Proceedings* 6.Suppl 3 (2012): O27.

Volek, J. S., et al. "Comparison of Energy-Restricted Very Low-Carbohydrate and Low-Fat Diets on Weight Loss and Body Composition in Overweight Men and Women." Nutrition and Metabolism 1.1 (2004):13.

Volek, J. S., et al. "Modification of Lipoproteins by Very-Low-Carbohydrate Diets." *Journal of Nutrition* 135.6 (2005): 1339–42.

Volek, J. S., and S. D. Phinney. "A New Look at Carbohydrate-Restricted Diets." *Nutrition Today* 48.2 (2013): E1–E7.

Volek, J. S., S. D. Phinney, C. E. Forsythe, E. E. Quann, R. J. Wood, M. J. Puglisi, W. J. Kraemer, D. M. Bibus, M. L. Fernandez, and R. D. Feinman. "Carbohydrate Restriction Has a More Favorable Impact on the Metabolic Syndrome than a Low-Fat Diet." *Lipids* 44.4 (2009): 297–309.

Volek, J. S., S. D. Phinney, E. Kossoff, J. A. Eberstein, and J. Moore. *The Art and Science of Low Carbohydrate Living: An Expert Guide to Making the Life-Saving Benefits of Carbohydrate Restriction Sustainable and Enjoyable.* Lexington, KY: Beyond Obesity, 2011.

Volek, J. S., E. E. Quann, and C. E. Forsythe. "Low-Carbohydrate Diets Promote a More Favorable Body Composition Than Low-Fat Diets." *Strength and Conditioning Journal* 32.1 (2010): 42–47.

Volek, J. S., and M. J. Sharman. "Cardiovascular and Hormonal Aspects of Very-Low-Carbohydrate Ketogenic Diets." *Obesity* 12 (2004): 115S–123S.

"Volek, J. and Phinney, "The Sad Saga of Saturated Fat–Low Carb Friends." http://www.lowcarbfriends.com/bbs/recommended-reading/805881-volek-phinney-sad-saga-saturated-fat.html.

Warshaw, H. S., and K. M. Bolderman. *Practical Carbohydrate Counting: A How-to-Teach Guide for Health Professionals.* Alexandria, VA: American Diabetes Association, 2008.

Weinstock, L. B., C. G. Klutke, and H. C. Lin. "Small Intestinal Bacterial Overgrowth in Patients with Interstitial Cystitis and Gastrointestinal Symptoms." *Digestive Diseases and Sciences* 53.5 (2008): 1246–51.

Weinstock, L. B., and A. S. Walters. "Restless Legs Syndrome Is Associated with Irritable Bowel Syndrome and Small Intestinal Bacterial Overgrowth." *Sleep Medicine* 12.6 (2011): 610–13.

West, R., M. S. Beeri, J. Schmeidler, C. M. Hannigan, G. Angelo, H. T. Grossman, C. Rosendorff, and J. M. Silverman. "Better Memory Functioning Associated with Higher Total and Low-Density Lipoprotein Cholesterol Levels in Very Elderly Subjects without the Apolipoprotein E4 Allele." *American Journal of Geriatric Psychiatry* 16.9 (2008): 781–85.

Westman, E. C. "Is Dietary Carbohydrate Essential for Human Nutrition?" *American Society for Clinical Nutrition* 75.5 (2002): 951–53.

Westman, E. C., S. D. Phinney, and J. Volek. *The New Atkins for a New You: The Ultimate Diet for Shedding Weight and Feeling Great Forever.* New York: Simon & Schuster, 2010.

Westman, E. C., and N. J. Stone. "Is a Low-Carbohydrate Diet the Best Diet for Metabolic Syndrome?" *Internal Medicine News* 40.14 (2007): 11.

Westman, E. C., W. S. Yancy, J. C. Mavropoulos, M. Marquart, and J. R. McDuffie. "The Effect of a Low-Carbohydrate, Ketogenic Diet versus a Low-Glycemic Index Diet on Glycemic Control in Type 2 Diabetes Mellitus." *Nutrition & Metabolism* 5.1 (2008): 36.

Wolever, T. M., and K. Bhaskaran. "Use of Glycemic Index to Estimate Mixed-Meal Glycemic Response." *American Journal of Clinical Nutrition* 95.1 (2011): 256–57. Web.

Wurtman, J. J., and R. J. Wurtman. "Brain Serotonin, Dietary Carbohydrates, Obesity and Depression." *European Neuropsychopharmacology* 2.3 (1992): 183–84.

Yamini, D., and M. Pimentel. "Irritable Bowel Syndrome and Small Intestinal Bacterial Overgrowth." *Journal of Clinical Gastroenterology* 44.10 (2010): 672–75.

Yang, X.-L. "Diabetes, Insulin and Cancer Risk." *World Journal of Diabetes* 3.4 (2012): 60.

Zhao, W.-Q., and M. Townsend. "Insulin Resistance and Amyloidogenesis as Common Molecular Foundation for Type 2 Diabetes and Alzheimer's Disease." *Biochimica Et Biophysica Acta (BBA)—Molecular Basis of Disease* 1792.5 (2009): 482–96.

Zioudrou, C., et al. "Opiod Peptides Derived from Food Proteins (the Exorphins)." Journal of Biological Chemistry 254.7 (1979): 2446–99.

Zlokovic, Berislav V. "The Blood-Brain Barrier in Health and Chronic Neurodegenerative Disorders." Neuron 57.2 (2008): 178-201.

# Index

abdominal obesity, 51
Academy of Nutrition and Dietetics, 105, 106
acellular carbohydrates, 33, 34
acetate, 100
Achilles carb, 41, 42
acid blockers, 77, 90
acid reflux, 70, 90
active fat, 54
addictive substances, model for, 40, 41
adenosine triphosphate. *See* ATP
ADHD, 73
adipose tissue, 50
aerobic exercise, 61
aerobic glycolysis, 62
alanine transaminase, 82
alimentary canal, 73
alpha cells, 50
ALT. *See* alanine transaminase
Alzheimer's disease, 73, 120
American Diabetes Association, 24, 105, 106
amylase, 125–26, 128
amylopectin, 16
amylose, 16, 125, 128
AMY1, 125–26
Amy2, 125
anti-DGP-deanimated gliadin peptide, 85
antigliadin antibodies, 86
antigliadin antibody IgA, 86

antigliadin antibody IgG, 86
antioxidants, 62
anus, 73
A1C. *See* hemoglobin A1C
aspartate transaminase, 82
AST. *See* aspartate transaminase
asthma, C-section delivery and, 66
athletes. *See also* endurance athletes
    carbohydrates and, 51–52
    triglycerides' use by, 61
Atkins diet, 27
ATP (adenosine triphosphate), 30, 31, 62–63, 119, 123
autism, 73
autoimmune disease, 67, 90
avocados, 137

barley, 32
beans, carbs in, 26
BBB. *See* blood brain barrier
belching, 90
belly fat, 54, 55–56
benzoate, 89
berries, 137
beta cells, 50, 55
beta-glucan, 32
beta-hydroxybutyrate, 122–23
betaine HCL, 87–88
bile, 73
bingeing, 27, 40
biofilm, 89

# About the Author

Cindy Carroll is a registered and licensed dietitian, a registered nurse and a functional/integrative medicine practitioner. She completed her Bachelor of Science degree at the University of Maryland Dental School, her Nutrition Plan IV from Simmons College in Boston and her Master of Science in Nutrition from the Massachusetts General Hospital (MGH) Institute for Health Professions. Her postgraduate nutrition internship was also at MGH. Cindy completed nursing school at Middlesex Community College in Bedford, Massachusetts. She has provided nutritional consulting for over twenty-five years in a variety of settings and currently has a private practice in Bedford and Lexington, Massachusetts. Please visit her website at www.nutritiontofityou.com.

www.ingramcontent.com/pod-product-compliance
Lightning Source LLC
Chambersburg PA
CBHW020000290326
41935CB00007B/252